Physical Signs in
Dermatology
Color Atlas and Text

Part 4

Clifford M. Lawrence

Consultant Dermatologist,
Royal Victoria Infirmary,
Newcastle upon Tyne, UK

Neil H. Cox

Consultant Dermatologist,
Cumberland Infirmary,
Carlisle, UK

M Mosby-Wolfe

Copyright © 1993 Mosby–Year Book Europe Limited
Except © University of Newcastle upon Tyne illustrations **3.5, 3.20, 6.4, 6.5, 6.39, 10.48, 10.81, 10.82, 10.90, 11.3, 13.7, 13.37, 14.12, 14.26, 14.35, 14.37, 18.22, 18.23, 19.7, 19.18, 19.40, 19.41, 19.42, 19.47, 20.47, 20.60**.
Except © Durham Health Authority illustrations **13.33, 13.34, 15.13**.
Published in 1993 by Wolfe Publishing, an imprint of Mosby–Year Book Europe Limited.
Reprinted 1994 by Times Mirror International Publishers Limited.

Reprinted by Royal Smeets Offset B.V., Weert, Netherlands.

ISBN 0 7234 1679 6

For full details of all Times Mirror International Publishers Limited titles please write to Times Mirror International Publishers Limited, Lynton House, 7–12 Tavistock Square, London WC1H 9LB, England.

A CIP catalogue record for this book is available from the British Library.

Library of Congress Cataloging-in-Publication Data has been applied for.

18. Erythema and Vascular Disorders

Erythema

The interaction of different pigments in the skin was discussed in Chapter 3. Changes in redness are the predominant colour change in most skin disorders, although some pathological processes are purely related to other pigments such as melanin. Furthermore, most changes in redness are due to changes in blood flow rather than to altered blood constituents, and changes in relative amounts of oxygenated haemoglobin are generally secondary to altered flow.

Erythema is an increase in redness due to increased visibility of intravascular blood, and is therefore usually the result of vasodilatation (**Table 18.1**). In most cases the vessels contributing to erythema are not individually detectable on examination with the naked eye, but appear as a diffuse redness. **Telangiectasia**, which consists of individually identifiable vessels, is not necessarily associated with diffuse redness and is discussed later.

It is important to recognise that redness is a normal feature of all skin, even though it may be difficult to detect clinically in coloured or very pale skin. It is also important to realise that vasodilatation is a labile process, subject to various controlling mechanisms, and that detection of erythema is subject to even more variables. As these will affect the degree of erythema in both normal and pathological skin, some of the factors influencing erythema are listed in **Table 18.1**.

Table 18.1 Some factors influencing erythema.

External	Light source, observer's perception of erythema
Factors altering refraction	Topical applications (e.g. oils) Thickness and quality of scale, epidermis, and dermis
Vascular anatomy	Density, depth, tortuosity, anastamoses and shunting, vessel type (arterial, venous, capillary), state of vessel wall
Blood	Erythrocyte count and haemoglobin level Proportions of oxy-haemoglobin and others (deoxy-haemoglobin, methaemoglobin etc.)
Factors influencing vasodilatation	Body temperature (skin and core), posture, exercise (skin flow and competing muscle flow) Neurological (emotion, sympathetic nerves) Local effects (trauma, inflammation, pH, vasodilator metabolites) Tissue chemicals (histamine, catecholamines, prostaglandins, etc.) and drugs (pharmacological or idiosyncratic effects)
Other pigments	Melanin, haemosiderin, extravasated blood etc.

Important points in assessment of erythema

Shades of red

Table 18.2 Shades of red.

Shade of red	Examples
Bright 'scarlet' red	Campbell de Morgan's spots (**6.23**) Pyogenic granuloma (**10.53**) Flexural rashes, especially candidiasis (**5.15**) Erysipelas (**18.1**)
'Ordinary' red	Psoriasis (**8.5**) Palmar erythema (**18.10**)
Brownish-red	Bowen's disease (**8.14**) Seborrhoeic eczema (**18.2**) Secondary syphilis
Pinkish-red	Pityriasis rosea (**7.17**)
Violaceous/purple	Dermatomyositis (**18.8, 18.9**) Lichen planus (**8.19**) Lupus pernio (**5.2**)
Dusky/blue	Cyanosis, methaemoglobinaemia Vascular insufficiency Some angiomas (**18.3, 18.43**)

Whilst accepting that erythema is subject to a variety of influences, it is important to recognise that shades of red exist and that some disorders may be very typical in their predominant colour (**Table 18.2**). Some of these were also discussed in **Table 3.1**.

18.1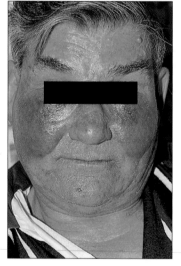

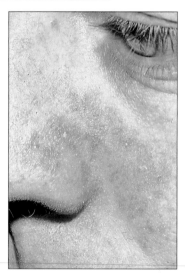 **18.2**

18.1, 18.2 Shades of red. Compare the beefy red colour of erysipelas (**18.1**) with the typically brownish-red colour of seborrhoeic dermatitis (**18.2**). Additional useful physical signs demonstrated here are the sharp demarcation and oedema of erysipelas, and the typical nasolabial fold distribution of seborrhoeic dermatitis (compare also with the more pink or violaceous red colour, and mid-cheek distribution, of lupus erythematosus, **18.5**).

Blanching

The physical sign of 'blanching on pressure' is not as absolute as standard dermatology teaching would suggest. Most common rashes have an erythematous component which, because it is caused by vasodilatation, will blanch on pressure. The presence of blanching, therefore, just confirms that erythema is present. Conversely, although lack of blanching on pressure may help to identify the presence of extravascular blood (*see* Purpura, p. 261), some localised vascular lesions are very difficult to blanch. The limitations of this sign are therefore as follows:

- Blanching of erythema is a feature of virtually all skin eruptions, so the presence of blanching has little discriminatory value.
- Some characteristically purpuric disorders also have a blanchable erythematous component, for example the

urticated lesions seen in Henoch–Schönlein purpura, which may lead to the assumption that the disorder is not purpuric.

- Some angiomatous lesions with purely intravascular blood are difficult to blanch with pressure (**18.3**). This may be because they are very small, and adeqate pressure cannot be applied to the relevant site without obscuring vision of the lesion. It may also occur because it is difficult to apply adequate pressure on soft areas such as the abdomen.
- Extravasation of fluid causes blanching of the associated vasodilatation in weals; these may not blanch further, yet are initially an erythematous disorder.

Even when correctly performed, this sign may be misleading as a mild degree of purpura is very common in inflamed skin, especially on elderly lower legs, in dermatoses which are not essentially purpuric (*see* **11.7**).

18.3

18.3 Superficial clustered angiomatous vessels can be difficult to blanch, and may resemble purpura.

Disorders characterised by erythema

Flushing

Flushing is a specific type of transient erythema, although frequent and prolonged flushing can be associated with fixed erythema or telangiectasia, for example in rosacea or in carcinoid syndrome. The most frequent sites are the face, upper trunk and upper arms, and the reaction occurs in everybody as a normal emotional response. There are, however, some local causes of flushing at other body sites also. Causes of flushing are listed in **Table 18.3**.

It is important to recognise that the cause of flushing is generally diagnosed by attention to the history and associated features rather than by physical signs in the skin alone, as these are indistinguishable from physiological flushing, except in disorders with additional fixed telangiectasia, e.g. carcinoid syndrome. The patient should be asked about drugs, alcohol and chemicals, and also other symptoms such as bronchospasm, gastrointestinal symptoms, headache, sweating.

Table 18.3 Causes of flushing.

Generalised	Physiological	Emotional, thermal, menopausal, hot foods
	Drugs	Alcohol (*see* below) Nitrates and other vasodilators, theophyllines, nicotinates, histamine, bromocryptime, tamoxifen
	Chemicals	Radiographic contrast media, inhaled solvents (**18.4**)
	Food additives	Nitrites, sulphites, monosodium glutamate
	Alcohol	*Physiological* Racial variation (especially Oriental races) *Interactions* Drugs: chlorpropamide, disulfiram Chemical: inhaled solvents (e.g. dimethylformamide, trichlorethylene)
	Pathological	Mastocytosis, phaeochromocytoma, Carcinoid syndrome, other peptide-producing tumours, hereditary angio-oedema
Localised	Physiological	Triple response to skin injury
	Facial	Fever, rosacea (**18.1**) Neurological abnormalities
	Acral	Erythromelalgia, resolving episodes of Raynaud's phenomenon

18.4

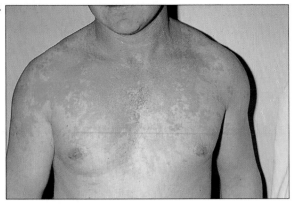

18.4 Flushing, in this case an exaggerated reaction following solvent exposure, is most pronounced on the face and upper torso.

Facial erythema

Childhood exanthemata

Facial erythema is a characteristic feature of scarlet fever and of erythema infectiosum (slapped cheek syndrome, *see* **11.9**). In scarlet fever, there is a typical circumoral pallor (*see* **11.10**); in erythema infectiosum there is a less prominent, but more specific sign which is reticulate erythema of the arms (**18.6**).

Butterfly rash

18.5

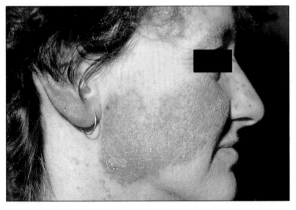

18.5 Butterfly facial rash of lupus erythematosus. This is much less common than other disorders which may produce a similar pattern (seborrhoeic and atopic dermatitis, rosacea).

This distribution of facial erythema causes one of the most frequent differential diagnosis problems in dermatology, mainly because one of the differentials, systemic lupus erythematosus, is potentially serious. The classic pattern is a rash on each cheek which extends across the bridge of the nose in a butterfly shape (**18.5**). Most patients with this pattern of erythema have rosacea, seborrhoeic dermatitis, other eczemas such as atopic or contact dermatitis, or transient erythema due to sunburn or systemic viral infections. Rosacea often affects the chin and forehead also, and has pustular lesions; seborrhoeic dermatitis affects the nasolabial area rather than the maxillary region, and is often at the browner end of the spectrum of red colours.

Localised rash

Localised areas of erythema on the face occur in many dermatoses, and the physical signs are not usually specific to the face. Red lips are a feature of Kawasaki disease (*see* **11.11**, **11.12**), often with red swollen palms and soles.

Reticulate erythema

Reticulate erythema describes a net-like pattern (*see* p. 22). It may occur as a physiological variant (*see* **6.21**), in livedo (*see* p. 257), transiently in some infections, or as a fixed pattern. Examples are given below.

Erythema infectiosum (Fifth disease, slapped cheek syndrome, parvovirus B19 infection)

A bright red 'slapped cheek' appearance (*see* **11.9**) is very typical of this disease. However, apart from being rather persistent and often occurring in an apparently well child, the appearance of this part of the eruption may be similar to flushing of the cheeks in any febrile child. The more specific part of the eruption is a striking reticulate erythema on the arms (**18.6**).

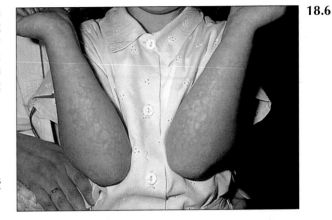

18.6

18.6 Reticulate erythema of the arms. The presence of this sign increases the diagnostic specificity of the 'slapped cheek' appearance of parvovirus B19 infection.

Erythema ab igne

Erythema ab igne is not uncommon. It is due to thermal damage to the skin and is usually found on the shins of elderly patients who sit close to a fire, although it can occur at other sites due to local application of heat, e.g. a hot water bottle (*see* **6.22**). Although initially red, there is a tendency to hyperpigmentation and hyperkeratosis, the latter having features similar to actinic keratosis. Development of pre-malignant or malignant tumours in affected skin is not uncommon. The pattern is basically that of the livedo distribution (*see* p. 257).

Genodermatoses

A reticulate pattern of erythema is a feature of some genodermatoses. A photosensitive tendency is often present also—although the reticulate erythema is an early and fixed feature, e.g. Rothmund–Thompson syndrome (**18.7**).

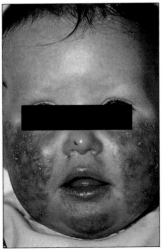

18.7

18.7 Reticulate erythema is a feature of some genodermatoses including Rothmund–Thompson syndrome, where the face is typically affected (*photo courtesy of Dr F. A. Ive*).

Streaky erythema

Dermatomyositis

A streaky pattern of violaceous erythema on the trunk is virtually pathognomonic of dermatomyositis (**18.8**), although other signs are likely to be present, and streaky erythema is not a requirement to make this diagnosis. The other prominent site of linear erythema, of the same violaceous colour, is along the dorsum of the fingers (**18.9**). The usual sign described on the fingers is smooth, purplish-coloured papular lesions over the dorsum of the joints (Gottron's papules), although rather more extensive linear erythema is actually more frequent.

18.8

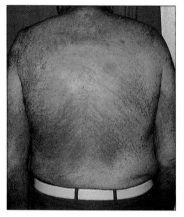

18.9

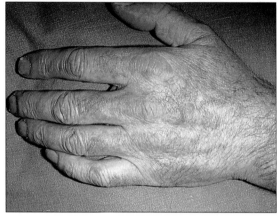

18.8 Dermatomyositis is characterised by a streaky pattern of violaceous erythema, which may resemble scratch marks.

18.9 Dermatomyositis. Typical purple-coloured lesions on the dorsum of the fingers, which form linear streaks and are associated with prominent nailfold telangiectasia and giant capillary loops (*see* **20.42**).

Palmar erythema

Palmar erythema can occur as a component of many skin disorders, but may also be the only site affected in some cases, such as psoriasis, contact dermatitis (*see* pp. 237–238), or dermatophyte infection (*see* **7.14**). In all of these situations there are additional physical signs, notably scaling, although this may be subtle in dermatophyte infection.

Red palms and soles are an early feature of Kawasaki disease in children; swelling and peeling occur later (*see* **11.11, 11.12**).

Palmar erythema without scaling occurs in several conditions; it may be relatively diffuse, but often most apparent on the hypothenar eminence (**18.10**). Gentle diascopy may reveal pulsatile flow.

Causes of palmar erythema without scaling include:

- Pregnancy and oral contraception.
- Hepatic disease.
- Thyrotoxicosis.
- Rheumatoid arthritis.
- Hyperglobulinaemia in other chronic diseases: leukaemia, bacterial endocarditis, obstructive lung disease.

18.10

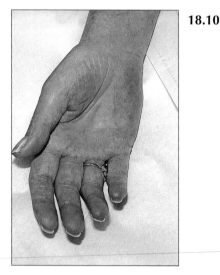

18.10 Palmar erythema is generally most prominent on hypothenar and thenar areas.

Other causes of erythema

Most rashes cause erythema to some extent. Maculopapular rashes are discussed in Chapter 11 and causes of erythroderma are described on p. 24.

Sunburn can affect any body site, and is noted specifically here because of the predictable time course of erythema. This develops about 6 hours after the exposure, peaks at 12–24 hours after a single insult, and fades with fine peeling.

Pallor and vasospastic disorders

Generalised pallor may be caused by anaemia, hypopituitism, or lack of sun exposure. The many causes of white skin lesions are discussed in Chapter 3. In this section attention is confined to vascular causes of pallor, listed in **Table 18.4**.

Table 18.4 Vascular causes of pallor.	
Physiological	'Vascular mottling' (*see* **6.21**) Cutis marmorata (*see* **6.20**), including an exaggerated congenital form
Occlusive arterial disease	Atherosclerosis, other (*see* later) (**18.39**)
Vasospastic disorders	Raynaud's phenomenon (**18.12**) Steal effect, and around many erythematous lesions (**18.11**); especially associated with angiomas and with psoriasis (Woronoff's ring)
Localised	Naevus anaemicus (*see* **3.16**)
Neurological	Migraine, Carpal tunnel syndrome (may cause early vasodilatation and later pallor or vasospasm)
Others	Weals (Chapter 17)

18.11

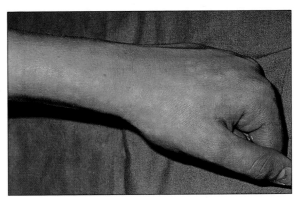

18.11 Steal effect. Localised vascular lesions, sometimes even quite tiny angiomas, often have a pale halo.

Raynaud's phenomenon

Raynaud's phenomenon is a clinically characteristic sequence of vasospastic changes, usually observed in the fingers. Vasospasm causes one or more digits to become white (**18.12**) or sometimes blue, followed by a period of dusky colouration, and often one of hyperaemia before returning to normal.

The important diagnostic features are:

- Variability: different digits are affected at different times and for different periods.
- Typical sequence of colour changes.
- Sharp cut-off from normal skin proximally.

The main differential diagnosis is **acrocyanosis**, which is a fairly common problem, presenting as pale or dusky-blue extremities in cold conditions. By comparison with Raynaud's phenomenon, acrocyanosis is less well localised, usually symmetrical, affects all fingers, fades out towards the wrist, has a slower onset and is more closely related to duration of cold exposure. It does not cause trophic changes, sclerodactyly, cuticle or nail changes, although these can all occur as a long-term consequence of Raynaud's phenomenon.

The causes of Raynaud's phenomenon are varied, and are outlined in **Table 18.5**. However, in many cases the cause cannot be diagnosed by the clinical features or by examination of the affected skin area alone; features at other body sites may help to establish a diagnosis (such as rashes of connective tissue diseases, livedo associated with hyperviscosity, evaluation of peripheral pulses and neurological features, etc.).

18.12

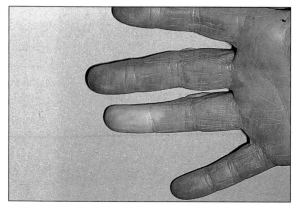

18.12 Raynaud's phenomenon is characterised by an extreme, sharply demarcated pallor.

Table 18.5 Causes of Raynaud's phenomenon.

- **Idiopathic**
  (Raynaud's disease)

- **Arterial**
  Compression
    Thoracic outlet disorders, trauma/fractures
  Occlusions
    Stenosis, thrombi, emboli, arteriosclerosis, Buerger's disease (thromboangiitis obliterans), small vessel occlusion in hyperviscosity disorders (*see* below)
  Collagen-vascular disease and vasculitis
    Systemic sclerosis/scleroderma, polyarteritis nodosa, lupus erythematosus, dermatomyositis, rheumatoid disease, Sjögren's syndrome

- **Neurological**
  Cervical spondylosis, compression syndromes, reflex vasoconstriction, hemiplegia and other chronic neurological disorders with disuse

- **Haematological**
  Hyperviscosity disorders (polycythaemia, cryoglobulinaemia, dysproteinaemia etc.)

- **Endocrine**
  Hypothroidism

- **Drugs/toxic**
  ß-blockers, nicotine, vinyl chloride, ergot derivatives, methysergide, heavy metals, bleomycin

- **Trauma**
  Vibration white finger

Livedo

Livedo is a specific pattern of impaired blood flow which is usefully considered at this point. The pattern is determined by the distribution of arterial blood supply to the skin, and relates to the fact that there is a relative 'watershed' area of slower flow between each adjacent area of blood supply. Thus, any disorder which slows flow further may make this watershed distribution more prominent, as the blood at this region is relatively hypoxic and more blue in colour. The livedo distribution has a reticulate pattern with a chickenwire appearance, often most marked on the lower legs. It may occur as a physiological response to cold, in association with abnormal vasospasm or with vascular inflammation. The latter generally causes more fixed patchy lesions known as 'broken livedo'. Some causes are listed in **Table 18.6**.

Table 18.6 Causes of livedo.

- **Physiological**
  Especially infants (**6.20**)

- **Idiopathic**
  Cutis marmorata (**18.13**)

- **Inflammatory vascular disorders**
  Polyarteritis nodosa (**18.14**), livedo vasculitis, leukocytoclastic vasculitis, other collagen vascular diseases

- **Vascular obstruction**
  Protein: hyperviscosity syndromes such as cryoglobulinaemia (**18.26**), macroglobulinaemia
  Erythrocyte: polycythaemia, sickle cell disease
  Crystals: oxalate, calcium
  Lipid: cholesterol or atheromatous emboli

- **Erythema ab igne (6.22)**

- **Drug-induced**
  Amantadine

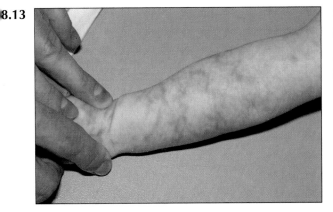

18.13 Cutis marmorata. A fixed livedo pattern with skin atrophy also, present at birth but often improving spontaneously during childhood (*photo courtesy of Dr F. A. Ive*). Compare with the 'broken' pattern of livedo in connective tissue disorders (**18.14**).

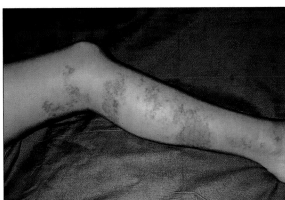

18.14 Polyarteritis nodosa with cutaneous livedo. The reticulate dusky discolouration is often patchy in intensity ('broken livedo').

Telangiectasia

Telangiectasia is the term used to describe visible small blood vessels in the upper dermis. The causes are listed in **Table 18.7**. Some of the more useful patterns and important causes are discussed below.

Table 18.7 Causes of telangiectasia.

- **Hereditary and genodermatoses**

  Hereditary benign telangiectasia
  Angiokeratomas, including Fabry's disease (**5.21**)
  Ataxia telangiectasia
  Rothmund–Thompson syndrome (**18.7**), Bloom's syndrome
  Xeroderma pigmentosa

- **Primary/idiopathic**

  Angiomas, angiokeratomas
  Vascular naevi, spider naevi (**18.15**) (also occur secondary to liver disease)
  Angioma serpiginosum
  Generalised essential telangiectasia
  Thread veins (**6.26**)

- **Secondary**

  Chronic vasodilatation
  　Sun exposure, varicose veins, rosacea, chronic bronchitis ('costal fringe')

  Hormonal/metabolic
  　Oestrogens, corticosteroids (exogenous or Cushing's syndrome),
  　carcinoid syndrome, mastocytosis

  Physical damage
  　Erythema ab igne (**6.22**)
  　Post-radiotherapy (**12.8**)

  Atrophic disorders
  　Poikiloderma (**1.16**), corticosteroid administration (**12.3**)
  　Necrobiosis lipoidica etc. (**12.9**)

  Connective tissue diseases
  　Dermatomyositis (**18.8**), scleroderma-related disorders (**12.33**)
  　Lupus erythematosus (**12.1**)

Physical signs of telangiectatic disorders

In many cases, the diagnosis of telangiectatic disorders is made clinically. To a certain extent, this will depend on factors such as age of onset, sex of patient, and family history; associated features of an underlying cause, such as diarrhoea and bronchospasm in carcinoid syndrome, may provide clues. However, the physical signs of the telangiectasia itself can be characteristic in several disorders, such as generalised essential telangiectasia, or may indicate a group of disorders, such as nailfold telangiectasia in the connective tissue diseases. Some of these are discussed below. There are also some useful general points:

- Telangiectasia will generally blanch with pressure, although this may be best directed to part of the lesion such as the central arteriole of spider naevi (*see* below). However, it can be difficult to demonstrate blanching in some tiny angiomas, possibly because the plastic strip or glass slide that is usually to hand is a crude instrument and does not provide the focal pressure required.

- Many angiomas and vascular naevi are oestrogen dependent so their apparent development during pregnancy is not an uncommon feature.

- Look at mucous membranes as well as skin, e.g. hereditary haemorrhagic telangiectasia.

The main patterns of telangiectasia are listed below.

Radiating pattern (spider naevus)

A spider naevus is a characteristic pattern of telangiectasia in which a central bright red papule, an arteriole seen end-on, supplies blood to radiating telangiectases. The resulting appearance somewhat resembles the handle and spokes of an umbrella. The diagnostic sign is blanching of the radiating vessels when the central, sometimes pulsatile and visibly raised, arteriole is compressed with a pencil point or similar implement (**18.15, 18.16**). The central pulsation may be made visible by partial compression using diascopy.

Spider naevi are seen frequently on the face in childhood and in teenage years, but can also occur in pregnancy, alcoholism, chronic liver disease (especially with portal hypertension), thyrotoxicosis, hereditary haemorrhagic telangiectasia (*see* **5.6**), and can also be related to oestrogen intake.

18.15

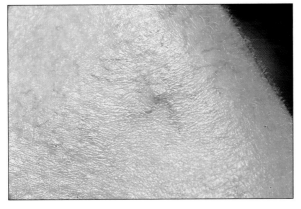

18.15 Spider naevus. This lesion is characterised by the central arteriole and radiating telangiectatic vessels; central pulsation may be visible.

18.16

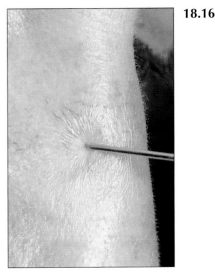

18.16 Spider naevus. The lesion can be blanched by point pressure on the central vessel (same lesion as **18.15**).

Focal grouped ectasias and matted pattern

18.17

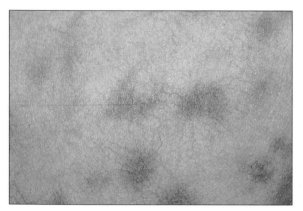

18.17 Telangiectasia macularis eruptiva perstans is a form of chronic cutaneous mastocytosis, in which a matted pattern of telangiectasia is observed.

Focal areas of telangiectasia occur in many conditions and are rarely clinically specific. The pattern is of multiple serpiginous vessels which appear to interweave; if enough vessels are visible this gives rise to a matted appearance. However, an obvious feeding blood vessel is not apparent, unlike in a spider naevus.

Small groups of vessels of this type are the most frequent type of telangiectasia in some naevoid vascular lesions, in scleroderma and in other connective tissue disorders. Similar, but smaller or less tightly grouped lesions can occur in radiation scars (*see* **12.8**), discoid lupus erythematosus (*see* **12.1**), rosacea and hereditary haemorrhagic telangiectasia (*see* **5.6**). Superficial small linear or serpiginous telangiectatic vessels are a feature of several discrete skin lesions, notably basal cell carcinoma (*see* **10.61**). Larger, more matted looking, lesions may be apparent in cutaneous mastocytosis (especially in the variant known as telangiectasia macularis eruptiva perstans, **18.17**), in Cushing's syndrome and in carcinoid syndrome.

Linear and arborising pattern

Tiny linear or wavy vessels, sometimes loosely grouped, are very common. They are often more blue than the types of telangiectasia discussed above, and are venous vessels, occurring on the upper back in young adults, on the legs—especially in women (*see* **6.26**)—around the costal margin of chronic bronchitic patients, and on the nose and cheeks in rosacea or chronic flushing.

More prominent lesions with a branching or arborising pattern are typical of generalised essential telangiectasia (**18.18**), and also occur in a more limited distribution on the lower legs as a frequent finding.

18.18

18.18 Arborising telangiectasia describes the linear branching pattern of vessels seen in essential telangiectasia. At a distance this resembles a sheet of erythema on the leg.

Punctate and papular pattern

Punctate or papular telangiectasia is seen in a variety of disorders, and some small ectatic vessels, or vessels viewed end-on, may appear as punctate lesions in many of the disorders already discussed. These are frequent in hereditary haemorrhagic telangiectasia and on the face in scleroderma.

More localised punctate telangiectasia is seen in radiation scars and atrophie blanche (**18.19**).

Small or early lesions in some disorders which are usually classified as angiomatous rather than telangiectatic may actually have the appearance of telangiectasia when viewed carefully. This is the case in patients with cherry angiomas (Campbell de Morgan's spots) (*see* **6.23**) and angioma serpiginosum (*see* **18.3**).

Angiokeratoma corporis diffusum (Fabry's disease) also falls into this category of small superficial ectatic vessels (i.e. telangiectasia) making up angiomas; this is an X-linked disorder which is therefore found in males. Lesions occur around the buttocks and genital area (*see* **5.21**), but can be widespread, and internal involvement in this condition affects vessels of the heart, kidneys, eyes and nervous system. It is due to an enzyme defect (α-galactosidase deficiency), and it is interesting that cutaneous angiokeratomas with a similar appearance and distribution have been described in other disorders with rare enzyme deficiencies.

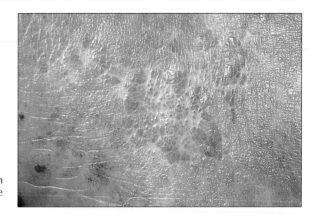

18.19

18.19 Atrophie blanche is a feature of venous disease in which punctate telangiectatic vessels with a scar-like appearance are visible in white areas.

Nailfold telangiectasia

Nailfold telangiectasia is one of the hallmarks of connective tissue diseases discussed in Chapter 20 and most prominent in dermatomyositis (*see* **20.40–20.44**).

Purpura and vasculitis

Extravasation of blood may present as bleeding, bruising (ecchymosis), and smaller purpuric lesions which are the most important dermatological manifestation of intradermal bleeding (**Table 18.8**). Tiny pinpoint purpura lesions are also known as petechiae. Most purpura is macular; palpable purpuric lesions suggest either a vasculitis or dysproteinaemia.

Ecchymosis or bruising is usually purple coloured initially and then changes to appear blue, grey, green and yellow. Bruises are most likely to be the result of physical damage to vessels by external trauma, but are occasionally due to clotting defects; they are less likely to have a dermatological cause than smaller purpuric spots. Further features which may help to determine the underlying defect are given in **Table 18.9**.

Before discussing the main physical signs of the skin lesions themselves, it is worth noting a few additional points in the examination of patients with purpura:

- Always consider symptoms or signs in mouth (**18.20**), joints, abdomen, eyes. For example, platelet disorders may cause bleeding from the gums, haemarthroses are a feature of some common clotting disorders, and Henoch–Schönlein purpura may be associated with joint pain or effusions and with colicky abdominal pain.
- Examine the eyes in all patients with purpura. In particular, vitreous or fundal haemorrhages suggest

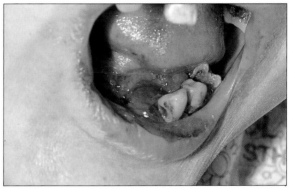

18.20

18.20 Haemorrhagic bulla of the gum in a patient with scurvy.

a significant thrombocytopaenic state and indicate a degree of urgency for diagnosis and treatment.
- Consider the importance of other skin findings, and assess whether the degree of purpura is out of proportion to the site and extent of associated skin disorder. This is discussed below with examples.
- Purpuric changes on the lower legs (*see* **11.7**) may occur in association with inflammatory dermatoses, especially in the elderly.

The main physical signs which are useful in the diagnosis of purpura are described below.

Table 18.8 Causes of purpura.

Decreased platelet number or function	Hereditary/congenital Idiopathic thrombocytopaenic purpura Other haematological disorders, e.g. leukaemias Increased consumption (large haemangiomas, hypersplenism, disseminated intravascular coagulopathy) Infections, uraemia, drugs and toxins
Vascular causes	Capillaritis and vasculitis (idiopathic, toxic/infective, drugs, systemic diseases) Altered connective tissue (age/actinic-related, corticosteroid, scurvy, lichen sclerosus et atrophicus, Ehlers–Danlos syndrome, amyloidosis Non-specific (minor feature in many dermatoses)
Other blood abnormalities	Dysproteinaemias Clotting disorders (usually cause bruising) Circulating anticoagulants

Table 18.9 Types of extravasation of blood related to underlying causes.

	Petechiae	Larger bruises	Bleeding (e.g. gums, joints)	Inflammation (i.e. palpable purpura)**
Underlying cause				
Coagulation defect	+/–	++	++	–
Platelet defect	++	+	+	–
Collagen defect	some e.g. scurvy amyloid	++	some e.g. scurvy	–
Vessel wall abnormality	++	+/–	some e.g. HSP*	++

– Not a feature.
+/– Not characteristic.
+ Frequent (but depends on severity).
++ Typical
*In Henoch–Schönlein Purpura (HSP) bleeding from gut wall may occur, but bleeding from gums is not a feature.
**Vasculitis may only be evident on histological examination.

Blanching

Purpura will not blanch under pressure, as it is due to erythrocytes in tissue rather than within vessels which can be compressed. As discussed above, this is not always a helpful physical sign. In purpuric disorders, it is important to remember the following points:

• An inflammatory component will blanch, so partial blanching may occur in vasulitic disorders or dermatoses of which purpura is a component.

• Lesions of capillaritis or resolving vasculitis may lose all their red colour when compressed, but still retain visible reddish-brown haemosiderin staining as evidence of previous extravasation of blood.

Variability

Purpura lesions are individually transient. They are bright red or purple initially, but become darker purple and later brown as their haemoglobin content is degraded to haemosiderin. This feature distinguishes them from angiomas which are fixed, and it is also helpful to determine if the process is ongoing. A good example is Henoch–Schönlein purpura, in which crops of lesions occur over a period of time, such that lesions of different age can be distinguished by their colour (**18.21**).

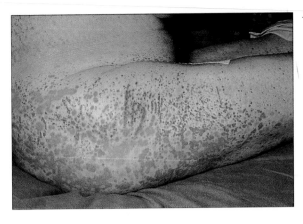

18.21

18.21 Henoch–Schönlein purpura, with lesions of different ages having colour varying between bright red recent purpura and brown haemosiderin of the earliest lesions.

Inflammation

Palpable purpura implies an inflammatory component rather than simple extravasation, although sufficient leakage of blood in thrombocytopenia may cause palpable lesions. In most cases, therefore, the presence of palpable purpura suggests the diagnosis of vasculitis, including dysproteinaemias. However, this is not necessarily true of deeper ecchymosis, in which the volume of blood in the tissues may be palpable as a diffuse swelling; it is also important to distinguish angiomas which may be palpable, but are fixed and do not fade over a period of time (*see* above).

Absence of palpable lesions does not exclude vasculitis as a cause of purpura, although subtle elevation of the lesions is usually apparent on careful inspection.

Patterns

Different patterns of purpura may be diagnostically useful and are therefore described below.

Linear

Purpura which is provoked by minor injury can appear as lines made up of many individual purpuric spots. If thrombocytopenia is excluded, then the cause is likely to be either a dysproteinaemia (*see* **2.34**) or altered supporting tissues of the dermal vessels (especially in amyloidosis, **18.22**).

18.22

18.22 Amyloidosis with linear cutaneous purpura after minimal trauma (pressure from bedding); the patient also had cardiac failure and macroglossia .

Circular/annular

Vaguely circular purpuric lesions, often including the lower limbs, are a typical feature in a group of disorders known as pigmented purpuric dermatoses (**18.23**). These are due to low-grade chronic capillaritis, and therefore exhibit petechiae at different stages. The background brownish-orange colour is largely due to haemosiderin, and a mild epidermal scaling component may also be present.

Performing the Hess test (*see* p. 55 may cause increased purpura within the lesions. The dusting of pinprick-sized orange-red purpuric lesions in these disorders is known as a Cayenne pepper appearance (**18.24**).

More sharply demarcated circular lesions, especially on the face, and with purpuric spots of a uniform colour, are strongly suggestive of artefact (*see* **16.42**).

18.23

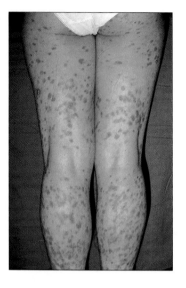

18.24

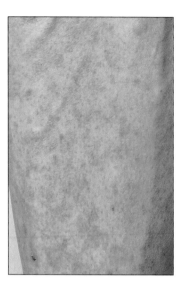

18.23 Pigmented purpuric dermatosis. The lower leg is the frequent body site for this group of disorders in which a low-grade capillaritis causes mildly scaling reddish-brown lesions with prominent haemosiderin content.

18.24 Pigmented purpuric dermatosis. Close examination reveals dusting of pinprick-sized haemorrhages, known as a Cayenne pepper appearance.

Reticulate

A reticulate pattern of purpura within individual skin lesions has been described as specific for vasculitis due to deposition of IgA immune complexes (Henoch–Schönlein purpura). This is a relatively unusual sign (**18.25**).

Rashes with an overall reticulate pattern may have an element of purpura which is in the same reticulate distribution. This occurs to some extent in erythema ab igne on the lower legs (*see* **6.22**), but is most important in the causes of livedo (seen in dysproteinaemias, **18.26**, and vasculitic disorders such as polyarteritis nodosa, cholesterol embolisation, etc., **Table 18.6**).

18.25

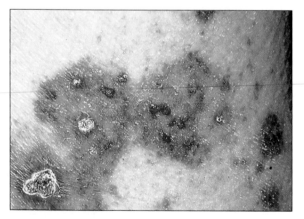

18.2

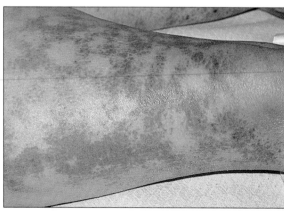

18.25 Henoch–Schönlein purpura. A reticulate pattern of purpura within lesions is said to be specific for vasculitis with IgA immune complex deposition.

18.26 Reticulate purpura in a patient with cryoglobulinaemia (*see also* **18.35**).

Overall distribution

Lower legs

This distribution is not very discriminatory, as most small-vessel vasculitic disorders are most apparent on the lower legs. However, the combination of lower leg and buttock involvement by palpable purpura is suggestive of Henoch–Schönlein purpura.

Head and neck

Fine petechial haemorrhages confined to the head and neck occur as a result of acutely raised intravascular pressure related to severe retching, coughing or the Valsalva manoeuvre. Because they occur at the same time, the purpuric spots are all of the same colour. This distribution is also frequent in amyloidosis, but in this there are also grouped purpuric spots related to mild injury and a more chronic course is apparent from the history and the presence of lesions of different colours.

Associated features

Connective tissue changes

Small sheets of purpura, with irregular edges, and often about 1–2 cm in diameter, are a common feature in thinned skin due to chronic actinic damage (*see* **6.13**) or as a side-effect of long-term or high-dose oral or topical corticosteroid treatment (*see* **12.3**).

Lichen sclerosus et atrophicus is a further cause of purpura related to connective tissue changes (**18.27**). The small (usually about 2–5 mm diameter) areas of purpura occur on a background of smooth, white atrophic skin. The main importance of this disorder is that it frequently involves genital skin in either sex and at any age, and the presence of genital purpura in children can give rise to concern about sexual abuse (**Table 2.6**).

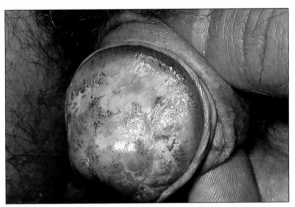

18.27

18.27 Lichen sclerosus et atrophicus. Altered upper dermal connective tissue alters the supporting matrix of blood vessels and is a cause of purpura.

Rashes

Purpura is a frequent component of many rashes. It may occur partly due to scratching, in which case it may have linear patterning and be associated with other signs of excoriation. However, it may also occur as a result of vasodilatation, especially on the lower leg (*see* **11.7**). In these situations, it is a matter of experience to decide whether the purpura is in proportion to the degree of inflammation and the general vascular status of the affected limb (**18.28**).

18.28 Purpura between ichthyotic scaling in a man with Hodgkin's disease. Purpura can occur in asteatotic eczema which is quite similar, but the amount of purpura shown here is out of proportion to the degree of scaling.

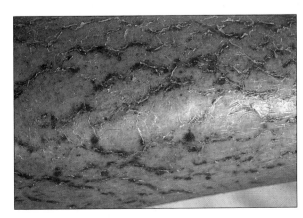

18.28

Urticated lesions

Urticated lesions are part of the spectrum of palpable purpura discussed above. They are especially frequent in Henoch–Schönlein purpura, but also in other vasculitic disorders. Purpura within urticarial lesions is also a feature of urticarial vasculitis (*see* **17.5**).

Follicular purpura

Follicular purpura is the hallmark of scurvy (**18.29**), although larger and deeper bleeding may occur and eventually cause 'woody' fibrosis. Other features which may be present include 'corkscrew' hairs (*see* **4.34**) which are actually multiply kinked rather than a spiral shape (*see* **6.3**), and bleeding from gums (**18.20**). It is important to note also that follicular eruptions, including purpura, are disproportionately frequent in HIV infection.

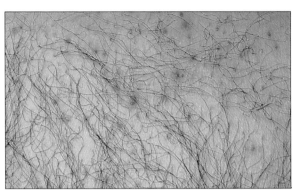

18.29

18.29 Follicular hyperkeratosis and purpura in scurvy.

Splinter haemorrhages

Splinter haemorrhages (*see* **20.50**, **20.51**) are purpuric lesions which develop a linear shape because of their site under the nail. The most frequent cause is trauma, but the most important causes are related to embolic and vasculitic disorders such as subacute bacterial endocarditis. Note that there may be evidence of vasculitis elsewhere, especially on the digital pulps (Osler's nodes) (*see* **20.52**) and other areas of the hands and feet (Janeway's lesions).

Vasculitis

Several signs of vasculitis have already been discussed in relation to purpura. However, vasculitis can cause many other types of lesion including pustules, necrosis, livedo, inflammation of fat, and so forth. Problems which arise when considering vasculitis include:

(a) Many causes produce clinically similar patterns.
(b) Both clinical pattern and histological features may vary during the course of a vasculitic process, and may be altered by non-specific factors such as localisation to areas of vascular stasis.
(c) Physical signs may be very variable, depending in part on the speed and degree of tissue anoxia. For example, temporal arteritis may cause extensive ulceration of the scalp (**13.27**), but generally does not cause any obvious cutaneous abnormality.
(d) Some vasculitic disorders are characterised by lesions which do not overtly suggest a vascular aetiology. For example, the destructive vasculitis of Wegener's granulomatosis, or the small scaling papules of pityriasis lichenoides (**18.32**).
(d) The situation is further confused by the wide range of different classifications of vasculitis, which may be based on clinical features, presumed aetiology, or histological features, such as size of vessels affected and types of inflammatory cells present. These are all useful in different ways:

• Clinical pattern classification is useful when faced with a patient with vasculitic lesions, but few patterns are 100% specific.
• Classification by cause is especially useful as a memory jog for the tests which may need to be performed in patients with vasculitis, but does not encourage a selective approach to investigation of individual cases.
• Classification by immunological mechanism is useful from a scientific point of view, but does not always translate easily into a clinically useful form.
• Classification by histological features is useful, and may help to predict outcome. For example, granulomatous vasculitis is generally more destructive than lymphocytic vasculitis, but the diagnosis is usually clinico-pathological rather than pathological alone.

As none of these is the single best way to divide up vasculitic disorders, a classification based primarily on known causes of vasculitis is given for reference (**Table 18.10**). The main text describes the different clinical presentations with a selected differential diagnosis for the various clinical presentations. Some lesions in which there is vasculitis, but which do not immediately suggest vasculitis on a clinical basis, are mentioned in more appropriate chapters. For example, pyoderma gangrenosum (*see* **13.18**) usually presents because of ulceration, pityriasis lichenoides (**18.32–18.34**) as papules, and so on.

Table 18.10 Causes of vasculitis.

Drugs	Blood products, sulphonamides, other antibiotics, thiazides, allopurinol, phenytoin, non-steroidal anti-inflammatory drugs
Infections	Direct vascular damage, syphilis, tuberculosis, infective ulcers/abscesses etc. Septic emboli Immunological reactions, meningococcus, gonococcus, viral
Arteritis and 'collagen vascular disease'	Wegener's arteritis, polyarteritis nodosa Churg–Strauss disease, giant cell arteritis Lupus erythematosus, rheumatoid disease Sjögren's syndrome, systemic sclerosis Behçet's syndrome
Other chronic disorders	Vasculitis associated with ulcerative colitis, cystic fibrosis, lymphomas, and 'tuberculides'
Thermal	Perniosis (chilblains)
Uncertain or multiple causes	Henoch–Schönlein disease 'Hypersensitivity vasculitis' Nodular vasculitis Urticarial (hypocomplementaemic) vasculitis Hypergammaglobulinaemic purpura Erythema elevatum diutinum

Clinical patterns

Clinical patterns of vasculitis may be quite varied. They are rarely specific, and a mixture of different patterns may occur in the same patient; for example, palpable purpura and cutaneous ulceration may be present simultaneously or sequentially. Additionally, some causes of vasculitis can give rise to a variety of clinical patterns; for example, sulphonamides may cause serum sickness, typical leukocytoclastic vasculitis, and erythema nodosum. Despite these limitations, it is useful to consider some typical patterns as they may help to narrow the search for a cause.

Palpable purpura

An eruption consisting of multiple palpable purpuric papules, most prominent on the lower legs, with each lesion generally about 5 mm diameter, is one of the most frequent forms of vasculitis (**18.30**). It is the hallmark of a small-vessel leukocytoclastic vasculitis (leukocytoclasia is the histological identification of fragmented neutrophil polymorphonuclear leukocyte nuclei in and around the damaged vessels). This pattern is seen in:

- Some drug eruptions.
- Collagen vascular diseases.
- Cryoglobulinaemia and other hyperglobulinaemic states.
- Henoch–Schönlein purpura.
- Associated with systemic infections.

Note:

- Urticated lesions can occur in any of these causes, but are typical of Henoch–Schönlein purpura; it is probably best to reserve the label of true Henoch–Schönlein purpura for cases with IgA immune complex deposition in vessel walls.
- Physical factors such as gravity (lower legs most floridly involved), pressure (e.g. tops of socks, **18.31**) and exercise may all enhance development of lesions.
- Pustules, necrosis, larger nodules and ulcers may all develop in any of the causes listed.
- Systemic malaise, arthritis, myalgia, nephritis and pyrexia may be a feature of any of the causes listed.
- Always suspect and exclude systemic infections and drug eruptions in patients with palpable purpura. Note that septicaemia can cause palpable purpura.

18.30

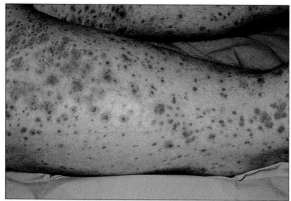

18.3

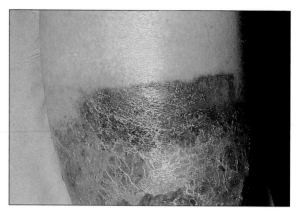

18.30 Palpable purpura, the hallmark of a small-vessel leukocytoclastic vasculitis.

18.31 Leukocytoclastic vasculitis with lesions accentuated by pressure from elastic in socks (*see also* **2.34**).

Other papular vasculitides

Papular lesions which are less obviously purpuric may occur in a form of lymphocytic vasculitis known as pityriasis lichenoides chronica (**18.32, 18.33**). This disorder consists of multiple brown papular lesions, generally about 5 mm in diameter, which may exhibit a shiny scale ('mica scale') on the flat-topped surface. Except in those individuals in whom a more acute and

necrotic version occurs initially (pityriasis lichenoides et varioliformis acuta, see below), it is more likely to be diagnosed as guttate psoriasis or a viral exanthem than as a vasculitis. Pityriasis lichenoides et varioliformis acuta (PLEVA) is an acute vasculitis seen mainly in children and young adults (**18.34**). Lesions are papular, haemorrhagic or necrotic and heal with scarring.

18.32

18.3

18.32, 18.33 Pityriasis lichenoides chronica. Small brown papular lesions which are not overtly vasculitic. Gentle scraping of the central papule shown in **18.32** has made the typical 'mica' scale more apparent (**18.33**).

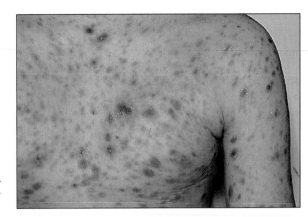

18.34

18.34 Pityriasis lichenoides et varioliformis acuta (PLEVA). The eruption is typically polymorphous and includes necrotic, papular and haemorrhagic lesions.

Pustular vasculitis

Pustules may develop in a leukocytoclastic vasculitis (*see* **15.19**). Consider also Behçet's syndrome (folliculitis-like pustules) or gonococcal vasculitis (relatively few, widely scattered, pustular vasculitic lesions with arthritis). *See also* Chapter 15.

Necrotic and destructive lesions

Necrosis may occur in many vasculitides, but is generally preceded or accompanied by either palpable purpura (**18.30**), inflammatory papules, or other evidence of a vasculitic process such as livedo. Haemorrhagic blisters may be a feature initially, followed by a hard black eschar of dead tissue (**18.35**). Similar haemorrhagic blisters may occur in some drug eruptions with a leukocytoclastic vasculitis, notably iododerma/bromoderma, and as part of the spectrum of pyoderma gangrenosum (*see* **15.20**). Infective pyoderma may be clinically similar.

In general terms, significant necrosis and destructive lesions are most likely to occur in granulomatous vasculitis e.g. Wegener's granulomatosis or lymphomatoid granulomatosis, or in vasculitis affecting large or medium arterial vessels e.g. polyarteritis nodosa. As usual there are exceptions; PLEVA is a lymphocytic vasculitis of small vessels but may be quite destructive (**18.34**).

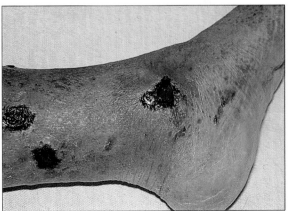

18.35

18.35 Necrosis in a patient with leukocytoclastic vasculitis. The dead tissue forms a hard black eschar. This was an exacerbation of disease in the patient with cryoglobulinaemia illustrated in **18.26**.

Nodular lesions and plaques

Nodular lesions and plaques may occur in conjunction with smaller palpable purpura lesions, but some specific patterns of nodular lesions with a vasculitic histology can be recognised.

Nodular vasculitis consists of purple nodules, often on the calf, which may ulcerate. This is really a descriptive label rather than a diagnosis; indeed, the term is often used for nodular vasculitic lesions where no other cause has been identified.

Erythema induratum (Bazin's disease) is a subset of this pattern which is associated with tuberculosis. Panniculitis is a deep inflammation of fat in which vasculitis may be either causative or a secondary feature. It generally presents as tender red inflamed nodules or plaques, frequently on the lower legs, and is generally less purple and less likely to ulcerate than a more superficial vasculitis. Causes of panniculitis in which vasculitis is an important feature include polyarteritis nodosa and thrombophlebitis. Lesions may produce deep tethering and a dimpled appearance as they resolve (*see* **12.36**).

Erythema nodosum is an acute lymphocytic vasculitis which affects dermis and fat. It causes multiple tender red nodules which are usually most prominent on the shins (**18.36**). It has many causes (**Table 18.11**).

Perniosis is a recognisable pattern of cold-induced lymphocytic vasculitis, again with involvement of the fat. It may present as lesions on fingers or toes, but is also relatively frequent on the lateral thighs in patients who are outdoors in cold wet weather (e.g. equestrian panniculitis, **18.37**). The lesions are itchy nodules, purple in colour, and the affected region of skin or the digits are often cold.

Sweet's disease (acute febrile neutrophilic dermatosis) is best considered here as it is characterised histologically by prominent neutrophil polymorph leukocytoclasis, although frank vasculitis is not a feature. It presents as acute nodules and plaques, sometimes triggered by upper respiratory tract infection, although the important association is with haematological malignancies and pre-malignancies (**18.38**).

Erythema multiforme is a lymphocytic vasculitis which may have a specific reaction pattern (target lesions, *see* **2.3**, **14.28**) but may cause lesions which appear more acute and overtly vasculitic. Plaques and nodules are the main feature, often with blistering due to epidermal necrosis and prominent upper dermal oedema. Lesions with typical target morphology suggest that the trigger is herpes simplex virus, but there are numerous other causes (*see* **Table 14.2**). It may be confused with urticaria, although non-specialists are more likely to diagnose acute urticaria as erythema multiforme than the converse.

18.36

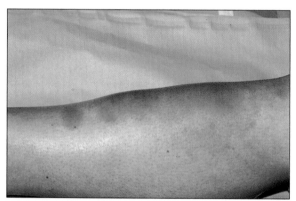

18.36 Erythema nodosum. Tender red nodules on the shins, not overtly vasculitic.

Table 18.11 Causes of erythema nodosum.

Infections	Streptococci Tuberculosis Yersinia
Drugs	Sulphonamides
Inflammatory	Acute sarcoidosis Inflammatory bowel disease
Neoplastic	Lymphomas

18.37

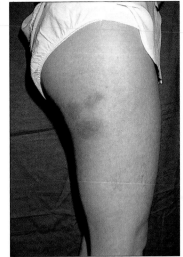

18.37 Equestrian panniculitis. This is a form of pernio (a cold-induced lymphocytic vasculitis). Lesions typically occur on the lateral thighs in horse-riders, and may also be seen in this distribution in children.

18.38

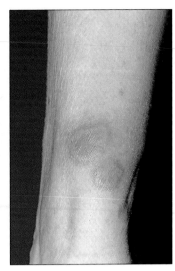

18.38 Sweet's disease. Acute inflammatory plaques on the arm with a characteristic yellowish-coloured bolstered edge due to intense infiltration with neutrophil polymorphs.

Stellate lesions

Acute meningococcal meningitis is the prime cause of vasculitic lesions with a prominent stellate pattern (*see* **2.10**).

Livedo

This pattern of vascular damage has been considered separately (*see* earlier in this chapter, **Table 18.6**).

Arterial and venous disease

Some causes and features of arterial and venous disease are described on p. 192. Arterial disease due to proximal atheroma, or where there is gangrene, tends to be the province of surgeons rather than dermatologists and is not discussed in detail. The features of arterial and venous disease are listed in **Tables 18.12** and **18.13**, respectively. However, it is important (especially with regard to treatment) to be aware that many patients have features of both; similarly, chronic venous disease and lymphoedema (*see* below) often co-exist.

Table 18.12 Clinical signs of arterial disease.

Pallor, cyanosis, poor capillary refill
Cool skin
Poor peripheral pulses
Atrophic shiny skin, loss of hairs
Dystrophic nails
Ulceration
Gangrene (**18.39**)

18.39

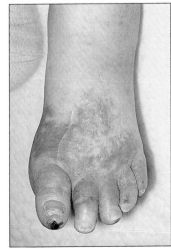

18.39 Arterial disease. Acute arterial obstruction causing pallor, reticulate dusky erythema, and gangrene of the tip of the hallux.

Table 18.13 Clinical signs associated with venous disease.

Varicose veins and 'venous flare'
Thrombophlebitis
Signs of deep venous thrombosis
Induration, lipodermatosclerosis
Shape change ('champagne bottle' leg)
Colour change (dusky, brown pigmentation)
Atrophie blanche
Cellulitis
Ulceration (Chapter 13)
Dermatitis

Venous obstruction

Venous obstruction may occur as a result of intravascular causes, e.g. thrombosis, vessel wall inflammation, or external compression, e.g. cervical rib tumour. The features are distal swelling, and pain in acute cases. The most important in dermatological differential diagnosis are deep venous thrombosis of the leg compared with cellulitis, and superior vena caval (SVC) obstruction compared with angio-oedema of the face. In SVC obstruction, the arms may also be swollen and chest veins are dilated (**18.40**). The usual cause is bronchial carcinoma.

18.40

18.40 Superior vena caval (SVC) obstruction. Dusky plethoric facies, oedema of the face and hands, dilated veins of the upper chest in SVC distribution.

Lymphoedema

Lymphoedema is not caused by abnormality of blood vessels, but of lymphatic vessels. It is appropriate to discuss it here as lymphoedema of the legs commonly occurs with chronic venous disease, and the physical signs may be very mixed. Causes and features of lymphoedema are listed in **Tables 18.14** and **18.15**. Although the condition is often stated to be non-pitting by comparison with other causes of oedema, this is not a reliable clinical sign. Although many lymphoedema states are chronic and associated with marked fibrosis, and hence a loss of tendency to pit on pressure, chronic venous oedema also causes fibrosis. Conversely, some degree of pitting can usually be achieved in lymphoedema.

Table 18.14 Causes of lymphoedema.

Primary

Familial, congenital, idiopathic
Associated with pleural effusions and yellow nail syndrome (**20.61**)

Secondary

- Infections
  Erysipelas/cellulitis (**13.31**)
  Other bacterial infections
  Granuloma inguinale
  Filariasis
- Iatrogenic
  Surgery
  Radiotherapy
- Neoplastic
  Tumour infiltration (e.g. breast, pelvic)
- Other causes of fibrosis
  Retroperitoneal fibrosis
  Chronic venous disease/lipodermatosclerosis
- Localised
  Pretibial myxoedema (**12.26, 12.27**)
  Rosacea (**15.11**)
  Tongue/lip (Melkersson–Rosenthal syndrome)

Table 18.15 Features of lymphoedema (**18.41**).

Swelling with limited pitting

Deeply bound down clefts between regions of oedema

Hyperkeratosis with deep fissures and warty changes ('mossy foot' or elephantosis verrucosa nostra*)

Nodules*

Secondary bacterial and dermatophyte infection

Association with yellow nail syndrome (Chapter 20)

*Late changes.

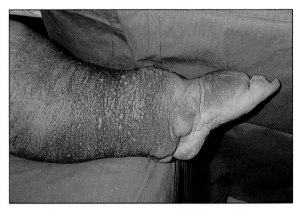

18.41

18.41 Lymphoedema. Massive oedema with typical tethering at the base of the toes and at the ankle (*see also* **7.28**).

Angiomas, localised vascular lesions, and vascular malformations

Some angiomas have already been described because they are likely to present as nodules, for example capillary angiomas (**10.54**), Campbell de Morgan spots (**6.23**), pyogenic granuloma (**10.53**), angiokeratomas (*see* pp. 145–146). Others have been discussed above in the sections on erythema and telangiectasia.

Three main areas remain:

- Superficial flat or plaque angiomas.
- Deep vascular malformations.
- Lymphangioma.

Superficial flat or plaque angiomas

Several benign and malignant vascular tumours may present as flat or plaque-type erythematous lesions, but are relatively rare, and often not clinically specific. Port-wine angioma is a recognisable pattern of malformation of blood vessels which has a dermatomal distribution on the face. It is typically a broad, flat, purplish red angioma (**18.42, 18.43**). Localised angiomatous nodules may develop in these lesions in older patients.

18.42

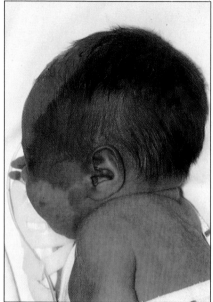

18.43

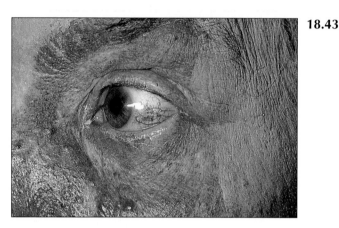

18.42, 18.43 Port wine stain. These are typically flat and red in colour at an early age (**18.42**) but may become a deeper purple and more palpable with increasing age (**18.43**). The importance of port wine angioma is an association with intracranial angioma (Sturge–Weber syndrome), and with conjunctival angiomatous vessels (**18.43**) and glaucoma (**18.42** *courtesy of Dr D. W. A. Milligan*).

Deep vascular malformations

Deep vascular malformations may present because of surface vascular changes or ulceration, but may also cause swelling or length asymmetry of limbs, venous dilatation, asymmetrical temperature of skin and other changes. Multiple nodular lesions may be associated with internal angiomas in the liver or gastrointestinal tract.

Lymphangioma

Lymphangioma may be huge and complex lesions, sometimes with other vessels also involved in a hamartomatous process, but the more common dermatological type is the lymphangioma circumscriptum (*see* **10.58**). They are described in Chapter 10, but are also included here since bleeding into the lesions is common, and they may be diagnosed as an abnormality of blood vessels.

19. Hair

Normal hair morphology and hair cycle

Body hair

There are major inherited differences in body hair distribution amongst normal individuals. The whirling pattern of body hair in dark-skinned children appears to follow the pattern of Blaschko's lines (*see* **2.8**).

The lower triangle pubic hair is present in men and women. Pubic hair above this line, sometimes referred to as the escutcheon, is present in men and approximately 10% of healthy females (**19.1**). Chest hairs are unique to males although periareola breast hair is common in females.

19.1 Normal female pubic hair. Ninety per cent of 227 healthy American women aged 18–40 years had a horizontal pattern, 9% the acuminate, 1% the sagittal and none the disperse pattern of pubic hair distribution. Almost 17% of normal men aged 30–40 years have the horizontal pattern of pubic hair. This distribution may be different in other ethnic groups. (From C. W. Dupertuis, W. B. Atkinson and H. Elftman (1945). *Human Biology*, **17**: 137).

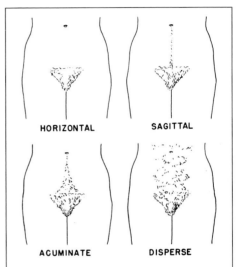

19.1

Hair cycle

A single follicle goes through several cycles of hair growth and rest in its lifetime (**19.2**). Normally 85–90% of all scalp hairs are in the anagen or growth phase, 10–15% are in the resting or telogen phase and approximately 1% are in the catagen or transitional phase. In the catagen phase, cell division in the hair matrix stops. The outer root sheath degenerates and retracts around the widened lower portion of the hair shaft to become a club hair. During the telogen phase, the non-growing hair is shed.

In the early part of the anagen (growth) phase, a new hair is produced which pushes out any remaining club or telogen hair. Between 50–100 of the 100,000 scalp hairs are shed each day.

Close inspection of normal scalp hair will reveal that many follicles have more than one hair emerging from a single follicular opening (**19.3**). On the scalp, hair grows approximately 0.4 mm each day (6 inches a year). The maximum length of the hair is determined partly by the growth rate, but more by the duration of the anagen growth phase. On average this lasts around 1000 days on the scalp, although anagen is longer in people who can grow their hair very long, and an anagen phase up to 8 years has been recorded. The anagen phase is much shorter in body hair, eyebrows and eyelashes.

19.2

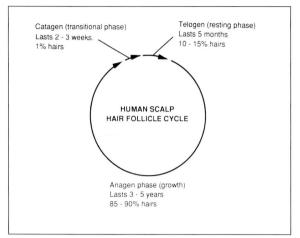

19.3

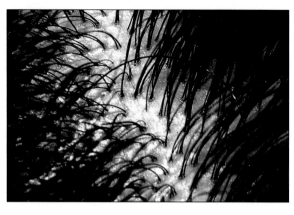

19.2 Hair cycle line drawing.

19.3 Normal scalp hair. On the scalp a single follicular opening is often shared by several terminal hairs growing from separate follicles. Close inspection of normal scalps will reveal that this is common, although most easily seen in people with diffuse alopecia.

Trichogram or forcible hair pluck

19.4

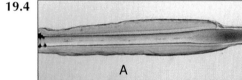

This test is used to determine the proportion of hairs in anagen or telogen, but is rarely used in clinical practice and remains an investigational rather than a diagnostic test. Using rubber-tipped artery forceps, a group of hairs, somewhere between 10–60 depending on the enthusiasm of the operator, are pulled out and looked at under a microscope. The proportion of telogen and anagen hairs (**19.4**) can be assessed from this sample and hair morphology examined at the same time. Artefactual abnormalities, such as extracting anagen hairs without the inner or outer root sheath, and fracture of an anagen hair, can occur.

19.4 Plucked anagen and telogen hairs. Anagen hairs (A) are firmly attached to their surroundings. When forcibly pulled out the normal anatomy is usually distorted and hairs may vary in appearance depending on how much of the outer root and inner root sheath is attached to the hair shaft. The dermal papilla and fibrous sheath usually remain behind. Shed telogen hairs (T) have the classic club hair appearance. Plucked telogen hairs may have an epithelial sac covering the club root.

Hair types

Lanugo hairs are present only on the fetus *in utero* and disappear at about 8 months. They are visible on premature babies as soft fine non-pigmented hairs (**19.5**).

Vellus hairs are fine downy hairs which cover the entire body surface except the palms and soles. Under the influence of androgens vellus hair will convert to terminal hair.

Terminal hairs are the thicker pigmented hairs found on the scalp, eyelash, eyebrow and secondary sexual hair.

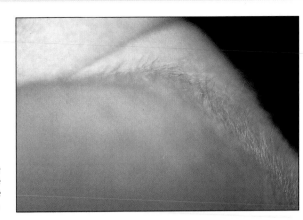

19.5 Lanugo hairs on a new-born infant. There are multiple small soft downy hairs visible on this baby's skin. This is the second growth of lanugo hair and is shed soon after birth. The first coat of longer lanugo hair is lost *in utero* at 7–8 months.

Increased hair growth

Hypertrichosis

Hypertrichosis is the growth of terminal hair, in a man or woman, at a site not normally hairy (**19.8**). This increased hair growth is not due to androgen stimulation, so other features of virilisation are not present. Hair growth may be generalised or localised (**Table 19.1**).

Table 19.1 Causes of hypertrichosis.

Localised	Congenital	Giant congenital naevus, pigmented naevi, Becker's naevus (**19.7**), naevoid hypertrichosis Spina bifida occulta—faun tail (**19.6**)
	Acquired	At the sites of constant rubbing or irritation, e.g. around leg ulcers, associated with chronic inflammatory disorders (**19.8**) Porphyria (**19.9**)
Generalised	Congenital	Sex-linked and autosomal-dominant generalised hypertrichosis Foetal hypertrichosis occurs in 10% of neonates with foetal alcohol syndrome
	Acquired	Drug-induced—minoxidil, diazoxide, cyclosporin A, phenytoin, systemic corticosteroids Anorexia nervosa and any cause of rapid weight loss. Porphyria cutanea tarda (**19.9**) Paraneoplastic (lanugo type hair)

19.6

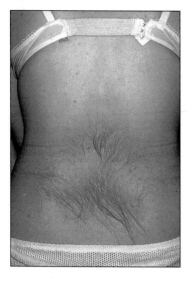

19.7

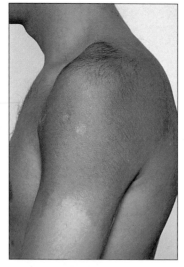

19.8

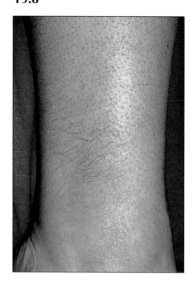

19.9

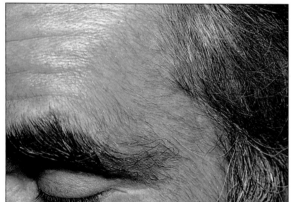

19.6 Localised hypertrichosis—faun tail. This is commonly associated with occult spina bifida (*see* **13.36**).

19.7 Becker's naevus. A common benign type of epidermal naevus with associated increased hair growth, that is more common in men and appears at puberty (*see* **10.25**).

19.8 Hypertrichosis after inflammation. Hypertrichosis may occur at sites of skin inflammation, e.g. around leg ulcers, and in this case after erythema nodosum. Repeated rubbing may also produce hair growth, e.g. on the shoulder in people who carry heavy weights.

19.9 Temple hypertrichosis. In the cutaneous porphyrias, hypertrichosis appears on sun-exposed sites. In this man, the cause was porphyria cutanea tarda.

Hirsutism

Hirsutism is the development of male pattern hair distribution in the female, caused by endogenous or exogenous androgens (**Table 19.2**). Coarse terminal hairs appear on the face (**19.10**), the male escutcheon and on the chest. Other signs of androgen-induced virilisation may also be present (**Table 19.3**).

19.10

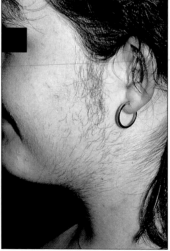

19.10 Facial hirsutism. Terminal hair growth is visible on the chin of this 40-year-old woman with idiopathic hirsutism. Increased hairiness at other sites, especially the thighs and abdomen, is usually also present.

Table 19.2 Causes of hirsutism.

Ovarian: polycystic ovary disease
Adrenal: Cushing's disease, virilising
  tumours, adreno-genital syndromes
Pituitary: acromegaly, hyperprolactinaemia
Iatrogenic: testosterone, stanozolol

Table 19.3 Signs of virilisation.

Absent or scanty periods
Acne
Reduction in breast size
Clitoral hypertrophy
Fronto-temporal balding
Deepening of the voice

Decreased scalp hair

Hair loss may be apparent as hair thinning or increased hair fall. In some cases hair loss
will also be associated with changes to the hair shaft.

Hair loss

Non-scarring alopecia

In non-scarring alopecia the follicle is intact, but does
not produce a viable hair. Non-scarring alopecia can be
diffuse, involving all scalp sites equally, or patterned,
where hair loss is localised to particular parts of the
scalp (**Table 19.4**).

Acute diffuse hair loss may be the result of anagen
or telogen effluvium (**Table 19.5**). Anagen hair loss
(**19.14**) occurs immediately after the insult, which is
usually iatrogenic and recognised by the patient.
Telogen loss is delayed by up to 3 months and the
precipitating event may not be immediately obvious.
Both must be distinguished from diffuse alopecia areata
by the absence of 'exclamation mark' hairs and other
features (*see* p. 281). Gradual diffuse hair loss (**19.15**)
is more common and usually idiopathic (**Table 19.4**),
although other causes must be considered.

Table 19.4 Non-scarring alopecia.

Diffuse hair loss	Patterned hair loss
Sudden onset Anagen effluvium (**19.14**) Telogen effluvium Diffuse alopecia areata	**Patchy** Tinea capitis (**19.40**) Alopecia areata (**19.19**) Secondary syphilis Trichotillomania (**19.39**)
Gradual onset Idiopathic (**19.15**) Endocrine: myxoedema, hypopituitarism Nutritional: iron deficiency Connective tissue disease: SLE, dermatomyositis (**19.17**) Infection: AIDS Diffuse alopecia areata	**Crown hair loss alone** Female pattern androgenic alopecia (**19.11, 19.12**) **Temporal recession with or without crown hair loss** Male pattern androgenic alopecia (**19.13**) Cutaneous viriliform in female **Marginal alopecia** Oophiasic pattern alopecia areata (**19.18**) Traction alopecia (**19.37, 19.38**)

19.11

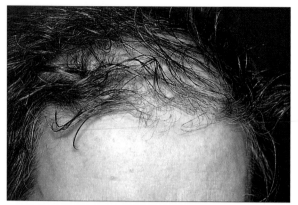

19.12

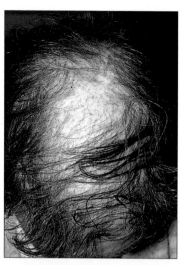

19.11, 19.12 Female pattern androgenic alopecia. There is loss of hair density over the centre of the scalp (**19.12**) with retention of the normal frontal (**19.11**) hair line.

19.13

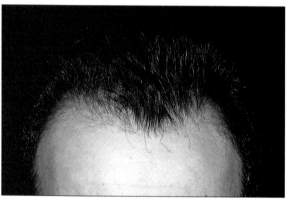

19.1

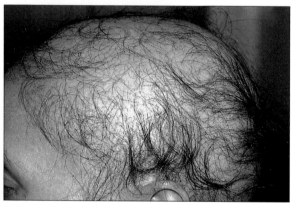

19.13 Male pattern androgenic alopecia. Initially there is temporal recession, followed by loss of hair from the crown of the head. Hairs at these sites become steadily finer before reverting to vellus hairs.

19.14 Anagen effluvium. This patient took 750,000 IU of vitamin A for acne. She developed weakness, exfoliation, blurred vision and loss of peripheral vision, followed by complete hair loss and her nails turned white.

19.15

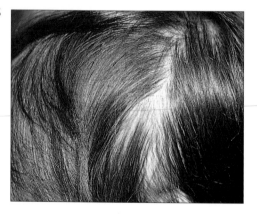

19.16

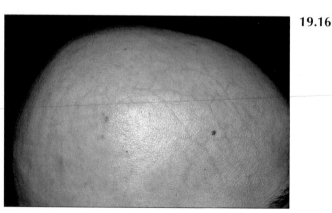

19.15 Diffuse hair loss idiopathic. There is diffuse hair thinning equally on the top and sides of the scalp. Compare this to **19.11, 19.12,** showing female pattern androgenic alopecia. This 22-year-old woman had a low serum iron, but did not respond to repletion of her iron stores.

19.16 Alopecia totalis. The scalp is completely bald. Hair follicle remnants are visible as tiny pits regularly spaced across the scalp. This is a type of alopecia areata.

Table 19.5 Comparison of telogen and anagen effluvium.

Telogen effluvium	Anagen effluvium
Occurs 2–4 months after the insult	1–4 weeks after the insult
20–50% of hairs lost	80–90% of hairs lost
Club hairs lost	Anagen hairs are lost with a pigmented bulb
No hair shaft abnormalities	Hair shafts may be narrowed or fractured
Causes	**Causes**
Acute, especially febrile, illness	Cancer chemotherapy
Childbirth (Hairs are maintained in anagen during pregnancy)	Poisoning by thallium, arsenic, vitamin A toxicity
Dietary	Radiation therapy
Drugs: warfarin, heparin, etretinate, carbamazepine, allopurinol	
Physical stress	

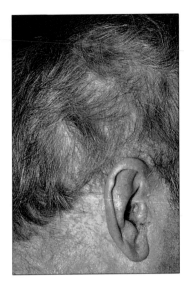

19.17

19.17 Dermatomyositis. In this man, who is also shown in **5.4**, dermatomyositis has caused diffuse scalp redness with generalised hair loss. This occurs in 20% of patients with dermatomyositis. Subsequent poikiloderma developing in affected areas may cause scarring alopecia.

Alopecia areata

Body and beard hair are commonly affected in alopecia areata. Complete scalp hair loss is called alopecia totalis (**19.16**) and complete scalp and body hair loss alopecia universalis. The oophiasic or marginated pattern of alopecia (**19.18**) is associated with a worse prognosis. Nail changes including fine pitting occur in up to 66% of cases (**20.17**). White hairs are usually not affected and this can produce striking colour changes as the pigmented, but not the white, hairs are lost in an individual with greying hair (**19.19**). Loss of eyebrow and eyelash hairs (**19.20**) can be disfiguring.

In alopecia areata, a poorly understood type of cell-mediated inflammatory reaction occurs around the hair follicle, damaging hair bulb cells and melanocytes and leading to hair loss and depigmentation. The extent of the inflammation around the follicle determines the type of damage seen in the hair.

Severe damage causes the hair to become dystrophic, enter telogen and break off. Hairs break because the keratogenous or hardening zone of the follicle, which is a few millimetres above the hair bulb, is also damaged by the inflammatory reaction, resulting in a weakened hair which breaks off just below the scalp surface. This leaves a dystrophic telogen hair remnant in the follicle. As this remnant is extruded from the follicle, the thin dystrophic and depigmented telogen hair root becomes visible at the follicle opening, with the normal-thickness remnant of the hair shaft above it producing the characteristic exclamation mark hair (**19.21, 19.22**). The associated absence of pigment in the tapered portion of the exclamation mark hair adds to the impression of tapering.

The inflammatory reaction on the hair root may result in virtual destruction of the hair remnant, leading to so-called cadaverised hairs (**19.23**). These black comedone-like plugs are visible in follicle orifices at the active margin, and can be expressed from the follicle using a comedone expressor. They are the degeneration products of the pigmented hair matrix, shaft and sheath and are considered to be a sign of aggressive disease with a poor prognosis.

Less severely affected hairs are also weakened at the keratinous zone, but not so severely that they break. These hairs can be made to kink when bent or pushed inwards, the kink corresponding to the shaft defect produced by the episode of alopecia (**19.24**). The kink gives the hair the shape of a coude catheter and the term coudability was coined for this sign in alopecia areata. This sign is either difficult to demonstrate or infrequently present. It should be looked for in normal-length hairs at the margin of a patch of alopecia areata where there are also exclamation mark hairs. Other less severely affected hairs are probably temporarily affected but do not break or go into telogen. The important conclusion to draw from this is that exclamation mark hairs are not always present in alopecia areata.

19.18

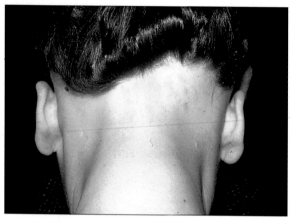

19.19

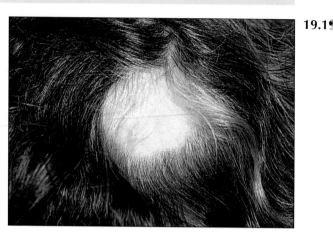

19.18 Marginal (oophiasic) pattern alopecia areata. Loss of hair at the temple, neck or forehead margins presages a poorer prognosis for regrowth than the patchy variety.

19.19 Alopecia areata patch of white hair regrowing. White hair is less commonly affected than pigmented hair in alopecia areata. Initial regrowth may be white hairs, and in patients with greying hair the depigmented hairs may be spared.

19.20

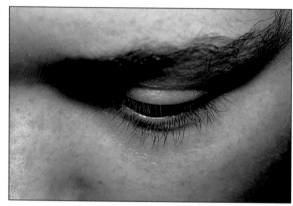

19.20 Loss of eyelashes in alopecia areata. Patchy loss of body and facial hair is common in alopecia areata.

19.21

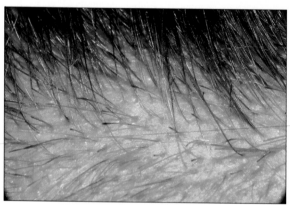

19.22

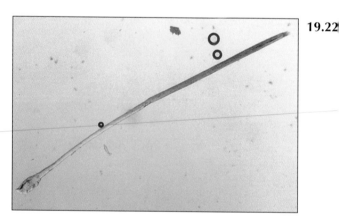

19.21, 19.22 'Exclamation mark' hairs. At the border of the bald area, exclamation mark hairs can usually be seen in active alopecia areata (**19.21**). The plucked exclamation mark hairs are dystophic telogen hairs with a tapered and depigmented base (**19.22**); note also that the broken end is ragged unlike the sharply cut-off end seen in trichotillomania (**19.39**).

19.23

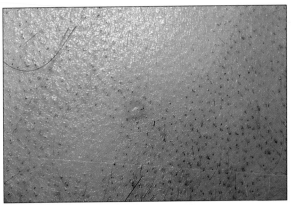

19.23 Cadaverised hairs in alopecia areata. There are multiple black hair remnants left in the follicles—the degeneration products of the pigmented hair matrix, shaft and sheath. These can be expressed using a comedone expressor, as has been done to a hair at the centre of the picture.

19.24

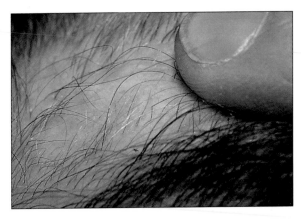

19.24 Coudability in alopecia areata. Less severely affected hairs are also weakened at the keratinous zone, but not so severely that they break. These hairs can be made to kink when bent or pushed inwards, the kink corresponding to the shaft defect produced by the episode of follicle inflammation.

Scarring alopecia

Hair loss resulting from destruction of the hair follicles may occur at any site, but is most noticeable in the scalp and beard. The bald skin is smooth, shiny and may be tethered or depressed (atrophic) compared to the surrounding tissues (**19.25**). Depression of the skin may also be present in alopecia areata; in this case it is due to loss of hair root substance in the bald areas compared to the surrounding hair-bearing skin. There may be signs of the active underlying disease within the intact hair at the edge of the bald area, for example the redness, scaling and follicular plugging of discoid lupus erythematosus (**19.26**).

Absence of visible follicles alone is not pathognomonic of scarring alopecia, since follicles may become almost invisible, e.g. in long-standing male pattern baldness. Commoner causes are listed in **Table 19.6**. Some of these are discussed below.

19.25

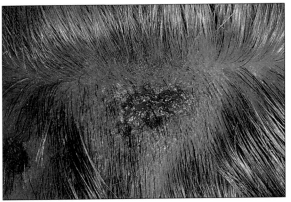

19.25 Localised scarring pemphigoid. Scarring or bullous skin changes without mucosal lesions may occur—usually on the scalp, forehead, or neck. In this case, there is just an erosion in the scalp which heals with scarring. Milia may also be present (*see* **14.30**).

19.26

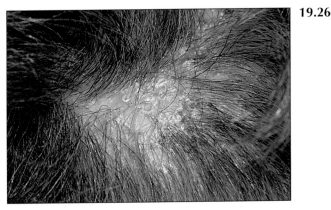

19.26 Scarring alopecia in discoid lupus erythematosus. Alopecia with loss of follicles and some residual inflammation at the periphery. This requires aggressive therapy whilst active inflammation is present in order to prevent irreversible hair loss.

19.27

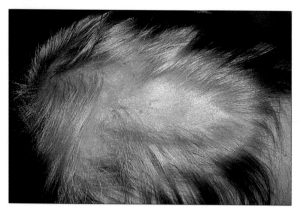

19.27 Cutis aplasia. Smooth shiny depressed scar tissue which is present at birth (ulceration may be present initially).

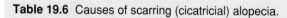

Table 19.6 Causes of scarring (cicatricial) alopecia.

- **Infection**
  Bacterial
    Pyogenic carbuncles, folliculitis, tuberculosis, tertiary syphilis
  Fungal
    Kerion, favus, microsporum canis
  Viral
    Herpes zoster
- **External Injury**
  Burns, trauma, radiotherapy (**19.28**)
- **Developmental**
  Naevus sebaceous (**10.45**)
  Cutis aplasia (**19.27**)
- **Neoplasms**
  Squamous and basal cell carcinoma (**19.29**) etc.
  Secondary deposits (**10.66**)
- **Inflammatory dermatoses**
  Discoid lupus erythematosus (**19.26**), lichen planus, dermatomyositis (**19.17**), scleroderma may result in the appearance of pseudo-pelade when the disease becomes inactive and only the damage remains
- **Blistering disorders**
  Cicatricial pemphigoid (**19.25**), porphyria cutanea tarda, epidermolysis bullosa
- **Idiopathic**
  Pseudo-pelade (**19.30**)
  Folliculitis decalvans (**19.31**)
  Folliculitis keloidalis (**19.32**)

19.28

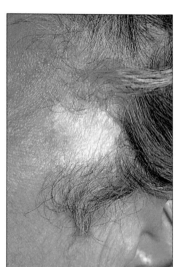

19.28 Scarring alopecia after radiotherapy. A patch of scarred alopecia remains at the site of radiotherapy for a basal cell carcinoma of the scalp.

19.29

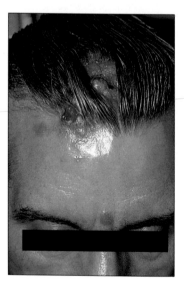

19.29 Squamous cell carcinoma of scalp. This man had a large and rapidly growing squamous cell carcinoma of the scalp causing hair destruction. The tumour had already metastasised at presentation. A skin metastasis is visible on the glabella.

Cutis aplasia

Cutis aplasia is a congenital absence of skin and subcutaneous tissue and is present at birth as a sharp marginated wound with a granulating base. Approximately 60% of cases occur on the scalp, at the vertex near the sagittal suture or over the parietal bones (**19.29**). The area usually measures 1–2 cm in diameter, but areas up to 9 cm diameter have been recorded. It is important to identify these as not being due to clumsy obstetrics.

Pseudo-pelade

Pseudo-pelade (pelade = alopecia) presents as irregular patches of scarring alopecia usually joined in a haphazard way, with isolated or groups of hairs remaining within the bald areas but no areas of folliculitis (**19.30**). The name was originally chosen because the appearance was considered similar to alopecia areata. Similar features are seen as an end-point of the inflammatory dermatoses (**Table 19.6**).

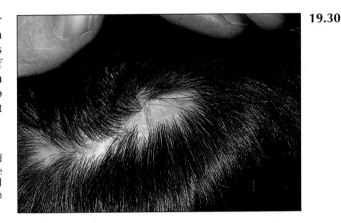

19.30

19.30 Pseudo-pelade. There are several oval or linear-shaped areas of scared alopecia with a very well-defined difference between the involved and uninvolved patches. The overall appearance has been graphically described as 'footprints in the snow'.

Folliculitis decalvans

Folliculitis decalvans (calvans = balding) presents as bald areas of scarring alopecia with follicular pustules at the periphery and bunches of terminal hairs left within the bald areas (**19.31**).

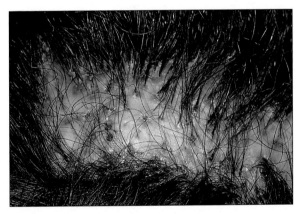

19.31

19.31 Folliculitis decalvans. Patchy scarred alopecia, in which hairs grow in bunches coming from a central follicular opening. There is associated folliculitis on surrounding follicles.

Folliculitis keloidalis

Follicular papules or pustules occur on the nape of the neck, particularly in Afro-Carribeans. The early inflammatory pustule gives way to a hard keloidal papule. These become confluent and a large keloid is left. Active pustular folliculitis is visible at the periphery (**19.32**).

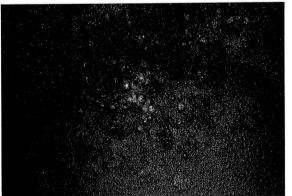

19.32

19.32 Folliculitis keloidalis. Follicular papules or pustules occur on the nape of the neck, particularly in Afro-Carribeans.

Hair shaft abnormalities

Hair shaft abnormalities, resulting in fragile hair that easily breaks, occur in a number of rare congenital anomalies and only the more common varieties are described here. Hair shaft breaks are also seen after mechanical damage or infection, and these must be distinguished from the exclamation mark hairs of alopecia areata (**Table 19.9**).

Monilethrix

Although inherited as an autosomal dominant trait, this abnormality may not become obvious until adolescence. The hair is thin, breaks easily and usually only short stubbly hair is apparent (**19.33–19.35**). Close examination of the hair shaft reveals the characteristic beaded appearance.

19.33

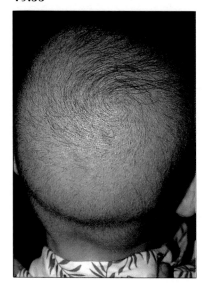

19.34

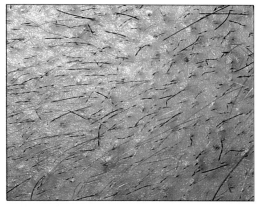

19.35

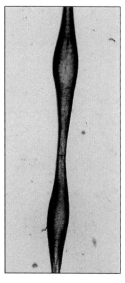

19.33–19.35 Monilethrix. The scalp is covered by multiple short and broken hairs (**19.33**). Closer inspection shows that the hair shafts are of uneven thickness (**19.34**), and the regular nodes can be clearly seen when examined under the microscope (**19.35**).

Pili torti

19.36

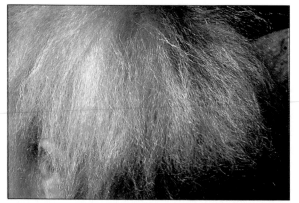

In pili torti, the hair shaft is flattened and twisted, giving it a spangled appearance, so that light is reflected from the hair shaft at different points depending on the position of the observer (**19.36**).

19.36 Pili torti. The hair is flattened and twisted around the longitudinal axis, resulting in each hair shaft assuming a spiral-like appearance and reflecting light at intervals along its length.

Trichorrhexis nodosa

Trichorrhexis nodosa is a common acquired cause of brittle or split-end hairs. Node-like swellings appear along the hair shaft, with fissuring or fractures at the site of the nodes. The hair cuticle splits due to repeated chemical and physical damage and the cortical substance ruptures out, producing a swelling or node on the hair shaft that is easily broken.

Mechanical damage

Traction alopecia

Repeated use of tight hair rollers, or a hair style that pulls hairs, such as a long pony tail or tight braiding (**19.37**) causes a permanent hair loss at the margins of the scalp (**19.38**). Initially there is an associated folliculitis around the affected hairs.

9.37

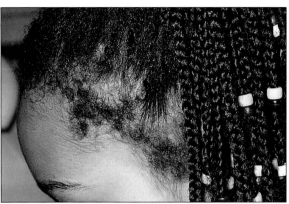

19.38

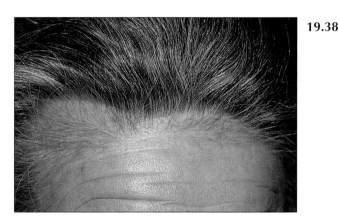

19.37 Traction alopecia in braided hair. Traction from plaited hair styles or long hair tied back may cause hair loss.

19.38 Traction alopecia marginal pattern. Repeatedly using tight rollers may lead to this type of marginal alopecia in which a few straggly hairs have survived.

Trichotillomania

This type of hair loss occurs when a disturbed patient consciously pulls out his own hair. Constant plucking or hair pulling leads to patches of hair loss, in which the remaining hairs are of various lengths but mostly shorter than 3 mm, since hairs shorter than this cannot be picked up with the fingers. There are no completely bald areas and the hairs feel stubbly when the palm is brushed over the scalp, as the broken ends are not tapered as occurs in normal hair (**19.39**). The broken hairs are still in the anagen (growth) phase and so are difficult to remove if plucked by the physician. By contrast, the short hairs of diffuse alopecia areata are all dystrophic telogen hairs, and come out easily when plucked with forceps. The broken root of the plucked hair can be identified with the naked eye. The area involved is usually sharply demarcated, on the crown or fronto-parietal region. Although the entire scalp may be affected the hair margin is commonly retained (**19.39**). Associated loss of eyebrow and eyelash hair is seen in approximately 25% of cases, so this is not helpful in distinguishing trichotillomania from diffuse alopecia areata. Some patients are said to swallow the plucked hairs and hairs may be found in the mouth or a hair ball may be palpated in the stomach.

19.39

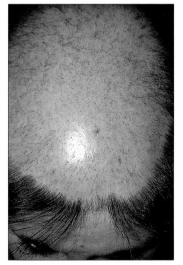

19.39 Trichotillomania. There is characteristic preservation of the frontal hair line. Hairs are mostly less than 3 mm long, and some scalp excoriations are present. Difficulty arises in cases where alopecia areata and trichotillomania co-exist (*see* p. 289).

Hair rubbing

Regular hair rubbing causes frictional damage and hairs break off near the scalp. This is most commonly seen in the lateral half of the eyebrow in children or adults with itchy facial eczema. In small babies who sleep on their back, a patch of hair loss and spangling of the hair shaft, producing a pseudo pili torti-like appearance, may appear over the occiput. In the first year of life, synchronised loss of telogen hairs from the occiput and parietal areas may result in temporary patterned hair loss at these sites (occipital alopecia of the new-born).

Other causes of broken hairs

Fungal infection (tinea capitis, kerion)

Fungi normally found only in man, the anthropophilic fungi, e.g. *Trichophyton tonsurans*, *T. violaceum* and *Microsporum audouinii*, produce little inflammation, as might be expected from a parasite in harmony with its host. These anthropophilic fungal infections may be of endothrix or ectothrix type (**Table 19.7**). Endothrix infections invade the hair shaft within the follicle, so the hair breaks off within the follicle and is seen as a black dot. Ectothrix infections grow on the surface of the hair shaft and invade the shaft only above the scalp surface, so that breakage leaves short (less than 5 mm long) hairs protruding from the follicle. The broken hairs may have a grey appearance due to fungal hyphae growing on the surface of the hair and these may fluoresce green under Wood's light (**19.41**, *see also* p. 53).

By contrast, fungal infections caused by animal ringworm, e.g. *T. mentagrophtyes* and *T.verrucosum*, produce inflammatory swelling in association with hair loss (**Table 19.8**). *M. canis* is an exception to this rule; this infection, usually acquired from cats, produces a well-circumscribed patch of non-inflamed hair loss (**19.40**).

Table 19.7 Patterns of scalp ringworm.

Clinical pattern	Hair appearance	Fungus	Fluorescence
Patchy alopecia, fine scale, little or no inflammation	Broken grey hairs (Ectothrix fungi)	M. audouinii M. canis	Greenish yellow* Greenish yellow
	Black dots (Endothrix fungi)	T. tonsurans T. violaceum	None None
Patchy hair loss, swelling and pustular discharge		T. mentagrophytes T. verrucosum	None None

*Although *M. canis* is an animal ringworm, in the UK it normally presents with non-inflamed scaly alopecia.

19.40

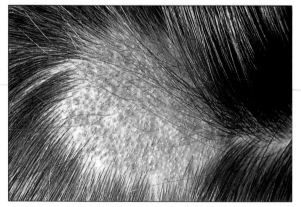

19.40 Tinea capitis. *Microsporum canis* infection caused a patch of alopecia with multiple broken hairs. There is no inflammation of the adjacent scalp.

Table 19.8 Likely animal* source in animal ringworm.

M. canis	Cat, dog, horse, monkey
T. mentagrophytes	Mouse, rat, dog, rabbit, guinea pig, monkey, cow, horse
T. verrucosum	Cow, horse

*Human to human spread can occur with all these fungi.

Differential diagnosis of extensive broken hairs

The clinical appearance of diffuse hair loss produced by diffuse alopecia areata and by trichotillomania can be almost indistinguishable, especially when exclamation mark hairs are absent (*see* above). Hair loss at other sites is not helpful, since this occurs in both conditions (*see* above). Furthermore, in some patients trichotillomania and alopecia areata may co-exist, although it is often difficult to decide which came first.

In both conditions, and occasionally in extensive fungal infections and congenital hair shaft anomalies, extensive broken hairs can be the principal feature. **Table 19.9** is an attempt to outline the clinical differences that may help in distinguishing these conditions. In general, broken hairs in alopecia areata are dystrophic and can be easily plucked out, and cadaverised hairs and kinkable or coudable hairs may be present. In trichotillomania, the broken hairs are all bristly anagen hairs that are difficult to pluck out, and there is no root depigmentation. Hair shaft abnormalities can be readily identified by careful examination of the individual hairs, although occasionally microscope examination is required. Fungal infections are normally excluded by fungal culture and potassium hydroxide microscopy, although the features listed in **Table 19.9** may also be helpful. It is important to recognise that absent fluorescence under Wood's light examination does not exclude fungal infection (**19.41**).

Table 19.9 Comparison of features of broken hairs.

	Alopecia areata	Fungal infection	Mechanical damage	Hair shaft abnormalities
Morphology of the broken hairs	Exclamation mark hairs or coudability	Dull grey or black dots hairs	Bristly hair, no completely bald patches	Beading, nodes or spangles visible on hair shaft
Plucking individual hairs	Easily removed	Easily removed	Difficult to pull out	Easily broken before removal
Appearance of the plucked hairs	Dystrophic telogen hairs	Fungal hyphae visible on KOH preparation	Normal anagen hair	Shaft defect visible
Trichogram of hair adjacent to the bald area	>50% telogen hairs	Normal (i.e. 10–15% telogen hairs)	100% anagen hairs	Variable

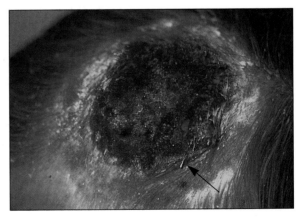

19.41

19.41 Fluorescence in tinea capitis. UV light examination of a patch of *Microsporum canis* alopecia. Greenish-yellow fluorescence is best seen on a single hair as indicated by the arrow. Only *M. canis* and *M. audouinii* regularly fluoresce with Wood's light. The fluorescence is seen only on the broken hairs, not on the surrounding scale. The trichophyton species, except *Trichophyton schoenleinii*, do not fluoresce, so Wood's light examination cannot be used to exclude fungal infection with these organisms.

Hair colour changes

In albinism and piebaldism (**19.42**), the hair is white from birth.

Acquired pigment change may be seen in pernicious anaemia and vitiligo, where patchy loss of pigmentation occurs. In alopecia areata, white hairs are less likely to be shed than pigmented hairs, so patients with generalised alopecia totalis and both pigmented and white hairs may retain the white but shed the pigmented and thus appear to go white-haired very rapidly (**19.43**). Cases of white hair turning grey have been reported in hypothyroidism. In kwashiorkor, loss of hair colour during periods of protein deficiency produces bands of light and normally pigmented hair—the flag sign; similar changes occur in protein deficiency due to gut disease.

External pigments also cause colour changes:

- Green. Copper from drinking water or industrial sources. Copper algicides used in swimming pool water.
- Yellow. Vioform medicaments. Nicotine staining.
- Orange. Dithranol stains (especially in grey or fair hair).

19.42

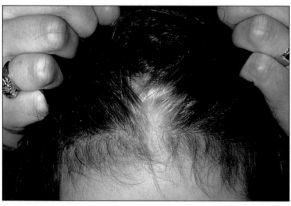

19.4

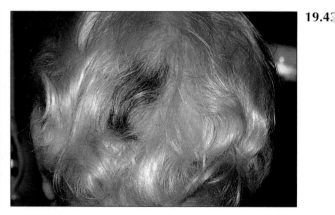

19.42 Piebaldism. The white forelock is characteristic of piebaldism, and a useful distinguishing feature from vitiligo. White patches in piebaldism are present from birth and often have hyperpigmented borders. **3.19** shows other features of the same patient.

19.43 Alopecia generalised white hair. This man developed almost total alopecia. The white hairs were unaffected as was a patch of pigmented hairs on the occiput, resulting in this remaining patch of black hair.

Additions to the hair

Small objects attached to the hair may be normal keratin peripilar casts or the egg cases (nits) left from parasitic infestations due to scalp, body or pubic lice. Peripilar casts, or scale due to inflammatory dermatoses (**19.47–19.49**) can be moved up and down the hair shaft, whilst egg cases are firmly attached to the hair. Adult lice can be identified with the naked eye as tiny insects holding on to the hair (**19.44**).

In the axilla, bacterial concretions collect on the hairs in *Trichomycosis axillaris* (**19.45,19.46**).

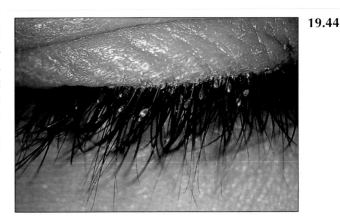

19.44

19.44 Pubic lice on the eyelashes.

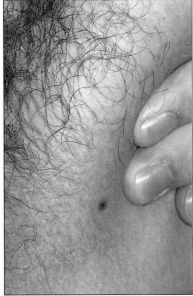

19.45

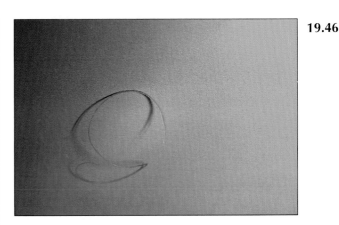

19.46

19.45, 19.46 Trichomycosis axillaris. Yellowish concretions of corynebacteria collect on the axillary hairs, producing an amorphous appearance of axillary hair and a thickening around the hair shaft. The portion of a plucked hair from within the follicle is relatively spared (**19.46**).

Scaling in the scalp

19.47

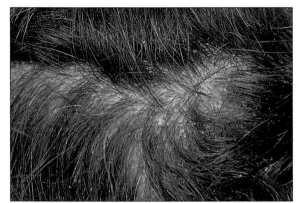

Scaling without associated hair loss occurs in a number of dermatoses. Fine diffuse scaling is due to dandruff or seborrhoeic eczema (**19.47**). Localised patches of well-defined scale separated by normal scalp is characteristic of psoriasis (**19.48**), and in pityriasis amiantacea (**19.49**) small adherent scales are formed through which the hair shafts grow, resulting in the hairs being stuck together by the scale. Because of this, hairs may be shed in clumps; single telogen hairs will not fall out of the adherent scale.

19.47 Seborrhoeic dermatitis of the scalp. There is a generalised fine scaling of the scalp. This is not raised and there are no spared areas.

19.48

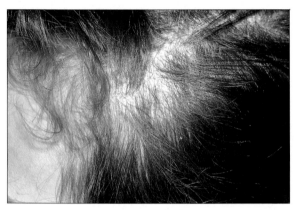

19.4

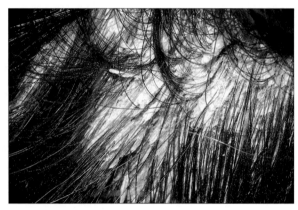

19.48 Psoriasis of the scalp. There is a well-demarcated patch of hyperkeratotic scale on this young girl's scalp with adjacent areas of uninvolved scalp skin. This is often better appreciated by feeling the scalp, when patchy hyperkeratotic plaques can be readily felt.

19.49 Pityriasis amiantacea. This may be the result of psoriasis or eczema. Adherent flakes of scale form on the scalp. The hairs grow through these, but as the scale is not shed the hairs remain joined together at the base by the scale.

20. Nails

Nail physiology

Fingernails grow approximately 0.5–1 mm per week, toenails more slowly. It takes approximately 6 months for a fingernail to grow from the matrix to the free edge and 18 months for a toenail to be replaced. Nail growth decreases with increasing age and poor circulation.Nail thickness increases distally because the nail bed contributes throughout its length to the thickness of the nail plate, adding a further 25% to the thickness determined by the matrix. The lunula (**20.1**) corresponds to the nail matrix. There is no adequate explanation for the white colour of the lunula, although this colour difference is apparent in both the nail plate and bed when the nail is removed.

The onychodermal band of Terry is the rim of pale nail, approximately 1 mm wide, visible at the distal end of the nail. It is often separated from the larger main pink zone of the nail plate by a thin white line. The nail bed just proximal to the onychodermal band appears more red than the remainder of the nail bed. Pressing the tip of the finger results in blanching of the onychodermal band and the proximal hyperaemic area more readily than the remainder of the nail plate. One explanation proposed for this observation is that this area has a different blood supply to the rest of the nail. Exaggeration of the colour differences in the onychodermal band has been recorded in cirrhosis, but similar changes are also seen in some normal individuals and it seems unlikely that this is a useful physical sign.

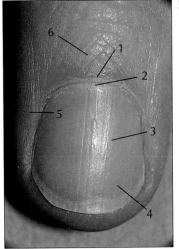

20.1

20.1 Normal nail showing the various parts: cuticle (1), lunula (2), nail plate (3), onychodermal band (4), lateral nailfold (5), posterior nailfold (6).

Normal variations and common anomalies

White flecks

White flecks (acquired punctate leuconychia) are common normal variants (**20.2, 20.3**). They are generally held to be incomplete keratinisation within the nail plate and appear to be the result of repeated minor trauma. They are not due to calcium insufficiency, a popular misconception. White flecks may disappear spontaneously or grow out with the nail.

20.2

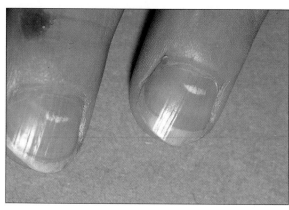

20..

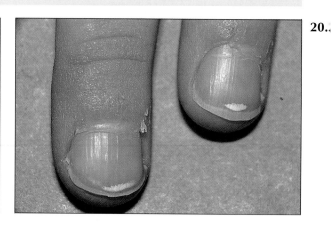

20.2, 20.3 White flecks (acquired punctate leuconychia). These appear to develop spontaneously but are probably due to forgotten mild trauma to the nail matrix. They are commonly curved and appear concurrently on several nails (**20.2**), usually in young people. Most disappear spontaneously before reaching the distal nail margin, while others grow out with the nail (**20.3**) as shown here 4 weeks later.

Longitudinal ridging

20.4

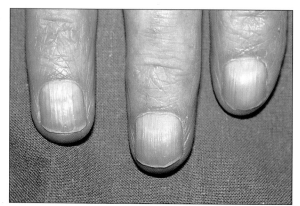

Longitudinal ridging becomes more obvious in old age. The ridges may appear beaded (**20.4**).

20.4 Longitudinal ridging. This is very common, but becomes more obvious with increasing age. Beading of the ridges also occurs. Longitudinal ridges in children usually point towards the centre of the nail rather than running parallel.

Shiny nails

20.5

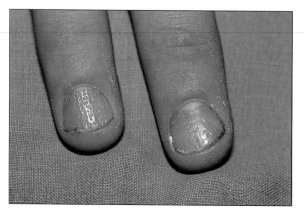

Shiny nails, due to rubbing, are commonly seen in long-standing itchy skin conditions (**20.5**). The free edge of the nail may also become bevelled with prolonged scratching.

20.5 Shiny nails and pitting in a patient with psoriasis. Nails commonly reflect back light when photographed and thus may appear polished. In these nails from a man with itchy psoriasis the rims of the deep psoriatic pits have been smoothed off by constant rubbing, producing an appearance similar to a well-polished brass name plate.

Pigmented streaks

Longitudinal pigmented bands are found in approximately 90% of Afro-Carribeans (**20.6**). The stripes vary in width from 1–7 mm and may be single or multiple. They are absent at birth and their number increases with age. The extent of pigmentation correlates with depth of skin colour, and in some extremely dark individuals nail pigmentation may be diffuse rather than linear. Histological examination shows that the streaks and diffuse pigmentation are due to melanin deposition within the nail plate.

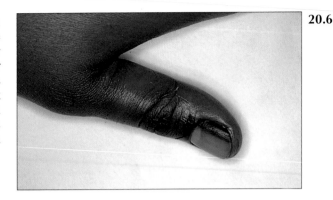

20.6

20.6 Pigmented streaks in black skin. A typical benign pigmented streak in an Afro-Carribean; although dark, the lesion had uniform width and was of long duration. Almost 90% of Afro-Carribeans have pigment bands and these are commonly multiple.

Congenital anomalies

Nail patella syndrome

The nail patella syndrome is an autosomal dominant trait. Patients have an absent or small patellae, prominent iliac horns (which can be felt but usually require X-ray examination to confirm their presence), and missing or small altered nails (**20.7, 20.8**). The nail changes are best seen on the thumb. A V-shaped lunula is the only feature on some nails and is pathognomonic. The importance of recognising these features is that associated renal anomalies, including glomerulonephritis, occur in approximately 30% of cases. Eye abnormalities including glaucoma also occur.

20.7

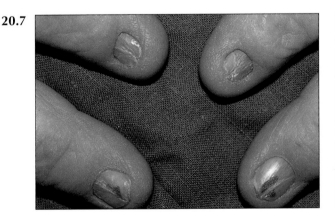

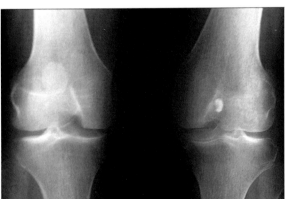

20.8

20.7, 20.8 Nail patella syndrome nails and X-rays of knees. Nails may be absent, small or split (**20.7**). Pterygium formation may occur and the triangular lunula is said to be pathognomonic and is usually best seen on the thumb. Bony changes include absent or small patellae (**20.8**), bilateral posterior iliac horns, hypoplasia of the capitulum and head of the radius. The clinically significant features are the associated renal and ocular changes.

Racket (racquet) nails

20.9

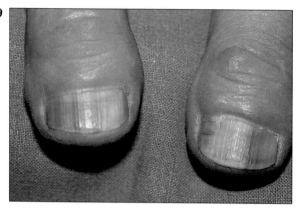

Racket (racquet) nails are shorter than they are wide and the terminal phalanx may also be short (**20.9**). In isolation, they have no significance. They are usually inherited as an autosomal dominant trait, but appear to be more common in women. They should not be confused with the finger shortening that occurs following reabsorption of the terminal phalanx in hyperparathyroidism.

20.9 Racket nails. These short nails are wider than they are long and were originally considered to resemble tennis rackets. The terminal phalanx is usually shorter and the big toe may be similarly affected. As an isolated finding this appearance is of no clinical significance.

Congenital malalignment of the toes

20.10

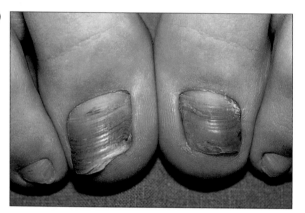

Congenital malalignment of the toes results in thickened nails (**20.10**) in children. These grow slowly, are generally very hard to cut, and usually malaligned so they do not grow straight. All the toenails are affected, but changes are usually noticed on the great toenail only.

20.10 Congenital malalignment of the great toenails. The nails are thicker and grow slowly, characteristically curving laterally with ridging of the nail plate. These changes can be readily distinguished from a fungal dystrophy, as the nail plate is formed from very hard keratin which does not crumble.

Trauma changes

20.11

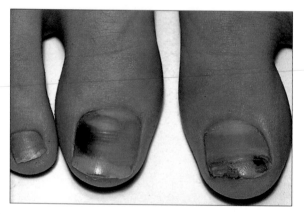

Repeated minor trauma to the toenails, due to poorly fitting shoes, ski-boots, tennis shoes, etc., causes black discolouration under the toenails due to subungual haemorrhage. There is associated lateral ridging, splitting, splinter haemorrhages and onycholysis. The hallux is the most commonly affected and the changes are symmetrical (**20.11**). In joggers, similar changes on the more lateral toenails have been recorded. Isolated subungual haematomas due to a single episode of trauma lead to discolouration of the nail bed. As the nail grows, the straight transverse margin defined by the cuticle can be distinguished (**20.12, 20.13**).

Handling solvents or oils can cause koilonychia, onycholysis and roughening of the nail plate (**20.14**).

20.11 Trauma changes in a footballer's great toenails. This condition usually affects the hallux nails and is bilateral in most cases. The nail is slightly thickened and distorted, with grey/green/brown discolouration due to bruising (*photo courtesy of Dr W. D. Paterson*).

20.12

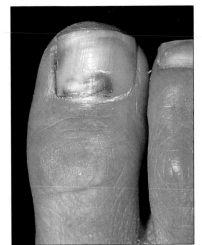

20.13

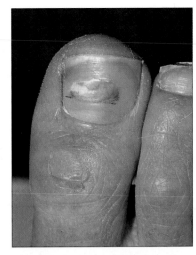

20.12, 20.13 Subungual haematoma in the great toenail. This can be distinguished from subungal melanin pigment because the colour includes red or purple, longitudinal spread of the blood is visible along ridges under the nail, and there is a sharp proximal border (**20.12**), which is initially just proximal to the cuticle, but becomes apparent as the nail grows (**20.13**).

20.14

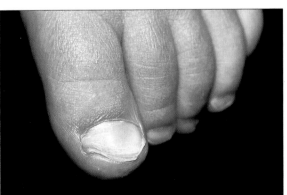

20.14 Oil-induced koilonychia. Abnormal nails in a motor mechanic. Repeated contact with oil and solvents lead to onycholysis mild koilonychia, with a roughened and discoloured nail.

Defects of the nail plate

Koilonychia

In koilonychia (hollow nails), the nails are spoon-shaped, and depending on the underlying cause may be thick, thin or normal (**20.15, 20.16**) (**Table 20.1**).

0.15

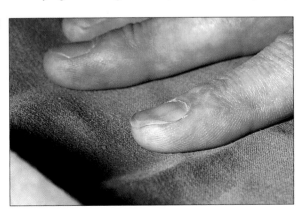

20.16

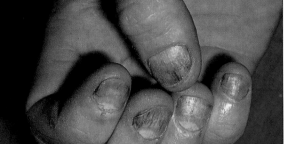

20.15, 20.16 Koilonychia (hollow nails). A single nail was involved due to trauma. Note the nicotine staining of the finger end (**20.15**). Most babies and small children have koilonychia of their toenails (**20.16**), and this is best seen on the great toe nail. It disappears spontaneously after about 4 years of age.

Table 20.1 Common causes of koilonychia.

- **Systemic**
  Congenital
    Autosomal dominant
  Haematological
    Iron deficiency with or without anaemia,
      polycythaemia, haemochromatosis
  Others
    Syphilis, endocrine disease

- **Local**
  Trauma
    Solvent injury, corrosive injury, thioglycate (acid
      perms used by hairdressers)

- **Cutaneous diseases**
  Raynaud's disease
  Lichen planus
  Alopecia areata

- **Physiological**
  In babies and toddlers, koilonychia of the hallux is
    common (**20.16**)

Nail pitting

Pits may be arranged longitudinally or horizontally, but these different patterns do not help with the differential diagnosis of the cause (**Table 20.2**). The morphology of individual pits can be helpful; pitting in psoriasis is well-defined and discrete, whereas eczema produces a shallower, or rippled pattern of pitting.

Table 20.2 Common causes of nail pitting.

Deep pits	Psoriasis (**20.5**)
Shallow pits	Alopecia areata (**20.17**)
	Eczema (**20.18**)
	Pityriasis rosea
	Syphilis

20.17

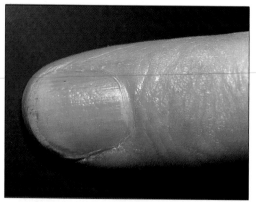

20.17 Nail pitting in alopecia areata. There are multiple tiny pits on the nail plate surface, producing a roughened appearance.

20.18 Nail pitting—eczema. Nail plate abnormalities occur as a result of periungual eczema. Here pits and transverse furrows have been created.

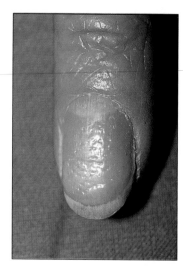

20.1

Clubbing

The soft tissues under the nail hypertrophy, and the nail becomes secondarily distorted (**20.19**). The normal angle between the posterior nailfold and the nail plate becomes flattened. A simple test for the presence of clubbing is to oppose opposite nails; in clubbing there is loss of the normal elongated diamond-shaped gap seen between the two nails, and at the proximal end of the nail there is a V-shaped gap. Some of the commoner causes are listed in **Table 20.3**.

<table>
<tr><td colspan="2">Table 20.3 Common causes of clubbing.</td></tr>
</table>

- **Respiratory (80% of cases)**
  Thoracic tumours: bronchogenic, pleural, lymphoma
  Chronic sepsis: bronchiectasis, abscess, empyema
  Pulmonary fibrosis: cryptogenic fibrosing alveolitis, asbestosis
- **Cardiovascular**
  Subacute bacterial endocarditis
  Cyanotic heart disease
- **Alimentary tract**
  Chronic liver disease
  Ulcerative colitis
  Crohn's disease
- **Congenital**
- **Endocrine**
  Thyrotoxicosis

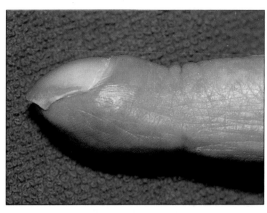

20.19 Clubbing. There is a swelling of the soft tissues under the nail, which pushes the nail plate upwards causing loss of the normal 180°, or less, angle made between the nail plate and the nailfold. The nail can be rocked on the underlying terminal phalanx by the application of gentle pressure.

Pincer nails

Pincer nails is usually a hereditary condition, although some cases appear to be due to wearing poorly fitting shoes (**20.20**). The transverse overcurvature of the nail plate may increase distally, so that the nail becomes cone-shaped or more pointed towards the tip. The residual area of soft tissue left between the distal pincers of the nail may become painful, due to compression of dermis and bone.

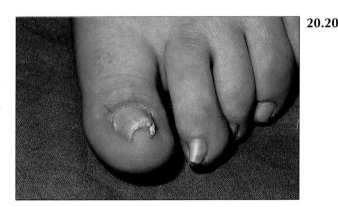

20.20 Pincer nails. This condition is usually most apparent on the thumb and great toe. The inward curved lateral borders cut into the nail bed and this is usually greatest at the free margin of the nail.

Thickened nails

Causes of thickened nails are listed in **Table 20.4**.

Table 20.4 Common causes of thickened nails.

Dermatological disease	Psoriasis (**20.21**), eczema, fungal infections
Old age	Thickened toenails are common in the elderly, probably due to impaired peripheral circulation (**20.22**)
Trauma	Onychogryphosis (**20.23**) is an extreme example
Congenital	Pachyonychia congenita

20.21

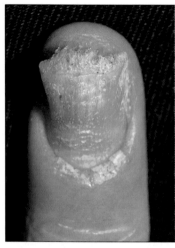

20.21 Thickened nail—psoriasis.

20.22

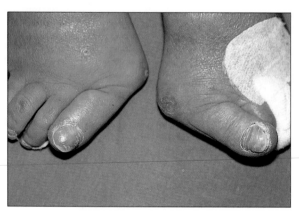

20.22 Ischaemic dystrophy of the elderly. Toenails are thickened, brittle and hard. Crumbly nails also occur, and if present a co-existing fungal infection must be excluded by fungal culture.

20.2

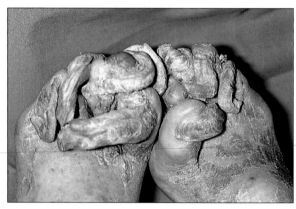

20.23 Onychogryphosis. There are a range of causes, including trauma, fungal infection and skin disease, causing thickening of the nails. Eventually the nail becomes too hard to cut and is left to grow unchecked, creating further trauma to the nail (*photo courtesy of Dr S. Natarajan*).

Nail ridging and Beau's lines

Ridges may be transverse or longitudinal; the latter are normal in old age (**20.4**). **Beau's lines** are transverse ridges which occur when nail growth stops temporarily, usually because of acute illness (**20.24**). In systemic causes, all the nails are affected at the same time, although because of differences in nail growth rates the changes will be seen first on the fingernails, in particular the middle fingernail—the fastest-growing nail, and lastly on the toenails. If the nail stops growing for more than 2 weeks, the defect in the nail is usually so great that the distal half is shed. Beau's lines are usually most apparent on the thumb and big toenail, probably because damage to these thicker nails can be greater without the nail being lost. Longitudinal ridging can result from a variety of causes (**Table 20.5**).

Guttering of the nail appears as a well-defined longitudinal groove of the nail plate, occuring due to compression of the proximal nailfold by a tumour, which is usually readily identifiable (**20.55, 20.56**).

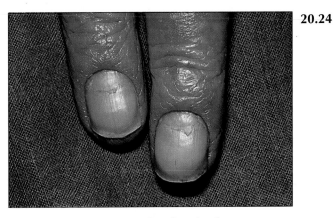

20.24

20.24 Beau's lines in drug-induced erythroderma.

Table 20.5 Types of nail ridging.

Longitudinal	Darier's disease (**20.25**) Median canaliform dystrophy (**20.26–20.29**) Physiological (**20.4**) Habit tick (**20.30**)
Transverse	Beau's lines (**20.24**) Eczema

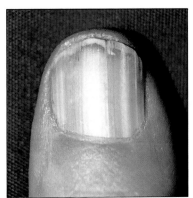

20.25

20.25 Darier's disease. White longitudinal streaks are common in Darier's disease. Where the streak meets the free margin there is usually a V-shaped notch. Nail splits and subungual keratoses also occur.

20.26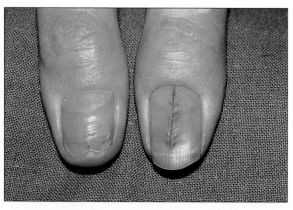

20.2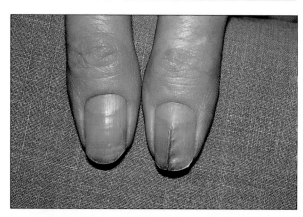

20.28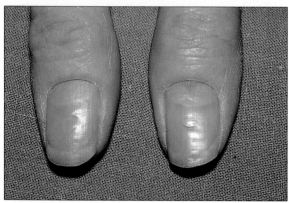

20.2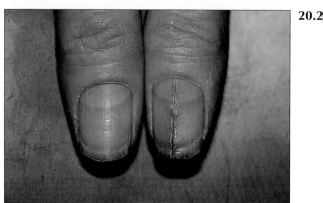

20.26–20.29 Median canaliform dystrophy. There is a central longitudinal fissure starting proximally (**20.26**). The same nails photographed 7 months (**20.27**), 20 months (**20.28**) and 36 months (**20.29**) later show spontaneous resolution followed by recurrence.

20.30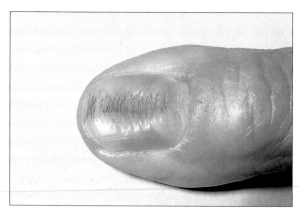

20.30 Habit tick dystrophy. Constant manipulation of the finger end adjacent to the matrix causes transverse ridges of the nail; as the nail grows serial ridges occur, and the final result appears as a longitudinal ridge.

Nail shedding

Nail shedding may occur due to trauma, severe acute illness, severe skin disease, drug reactions (**20.31**), radiotherapy or spontaneously (onychomadesis).

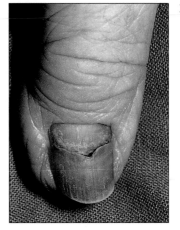

20.31

20.31 Nail shedding associated with an idiosyncratic reaction to azathioprine.

Rough nails

Changes to the nail surface producing roughness and opacity of the nail plate with splitting at the free margin occur in alopecia areata (**20.17**), psoriasis and lichen planus. The term 20 nail dystrophy was applied to such cases in which all the nails were involved (**20.32**). However, in childhood at least, histological changes in 20 nail dystrophy appear to be those of lichen planus.

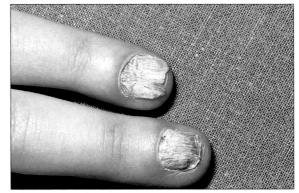

20.32

20.32 Rough nails—20 nail dystrophy. The nails may appear white with a mild surface roughness.

Flaky nails

Distal flaking of the free margin of the nails or brittle nails (lamella dystrophy) occurs in approximately 20% of the population. It is common in children and adults, and is the result of repeated trauma and immersion in hot soapy water or solvents (**20.33**).

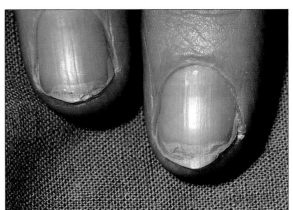

20.33

20.33 Flaky nails. The free margin of the nail is split into several layers. It is common in those who have a lot of contact with water and detergents.

Fungal infections of the nail

Fungal infections of the nail are usually the result of infection with *Trichophyton rubrum* and *T. mentagrophytes*. Three routes of dermatophyte infection which produce different physical signs are recognised; these become indistinguishable in advanced infections (**20.34–20.36**). Physical signs that may help with the differential diagnosis of nail fungal infections are summarised in **Table 20.6**. Candida nail dystrophy may occur secondary to ischaemia as in Raynaud's disease, following chronic paronychia, in chronic mucocutaneous candidiasis, or without an obvious cause (**20.37**). Causes of candida paronychia are listed in **Table 20.8**.

20.34

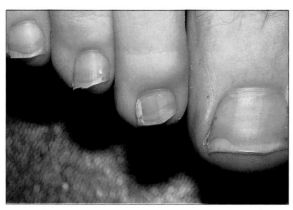

20.34 White superficial onychomycosis. Superficial invasion of the nail plate of the second toe produces patchy white change visible on the nail surface. The surface is soft, opaque and powdery and the whiteness can easily be scrapped away. The nail plate is not thickened. *Trichophyton rubrum* was cultured.

20.35

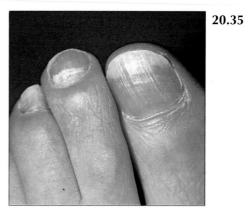

20.35 Distal subungual onychomycosis. Fungi invasion via the distal or lateral edge of the nail is common. The distal nail turns yellowish-white, thickens and crumbles, and starts to separate from the nail bed. *Trichophyton rubrum* was cultured.

20.36

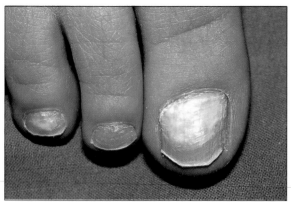

20.36 Proximal superficial onychomycosis. Infection occurs via the cuticle area within invasion of the nail plate. Hyperkeratotic debris collects under the normal surface nail plate, causing the it to separate from the nail bed. Transverse white bands may be seen. In this case *Trichophyton rubrum* was cultured.

20.37

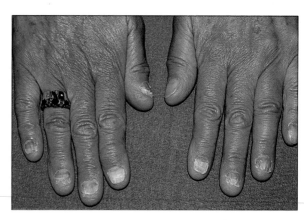

20.37 Candida nail dystrophy. Nine of this woman's fingernails were affected with koilonychia, thickening, onycholysis and splitting. All her nails returned to normal after a course of itraconazole. No predisposing cause was found.

Table 20.6 Differential diagnosis of fungal nail infection.

Psoriasis	Pitting (**20.5**) does not occur in fungal nail dystrophy. Salmon patches (**20.49**) do not present in fungal dystrophies. Asymmetrical involvement may occur in both psoriasis and fungal infections.
Leuconychia	Spontaneous white flecks can be distinguished from white superficial onychomycosis; the former cannot be scraped away since the whiteness is due to changes deep within the nail plate (**20.2, 20.3**).
Eczema	Secondary nail damage in eczema may produce horizontal ridging and pitting (**20.18**), but the nail remains hard and does not crumble.
Habit tick damage	The nail is deformed but the nail plate is normal and does not crumble (**20.30**).
Congenital anomalies	Pachyonychia congenita and congenital malalignment of the great toe (**20.10**) are usually symmetrical. Although thickened and deformed the nail plate is hard.
Ischaemic dystrophy of the elderly	Poor peripheral circulation causes thickening, roughness and sometimes onycholysis of the toenail plate (**20.22**). Secondary infection of candida can occur. The combination is predictably common in diabetics. Exclusion of a co-existing fungal infection requires fungal culture.
Trauma	Both big toenails are affected—particularly common in footballers (**20.11**).

Defects of the nailfolds

Ingrown toenail

In this condition, painful redness and swelling followed by the development of granulation tissue occur, due to a small spicule of nail penetrating the lateral nailfold (**20.38**). The spicule is formed by a combination of trauma, incorrect cutting of the nail and poor footwear.

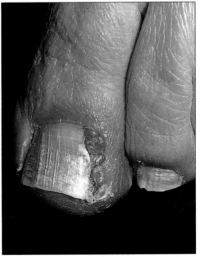

20.38

20.38 Ingrown toenail and associated nail plate fungal infection.

Pterygium

Scarring of the posterior nailfold skin and the dorsal matrix results in fusion of the posterior nailfold onto the nail plate (**20.39**). The nail may be completely eroded at the point of attachment and divided into two portions (**Table 20.7**).

Table 20.7 Causes of pterygium.

Lichen planus
Chronic ischaemia
Trauma
Nail patella syndrome
Dystrophic epidermolysis bullosa

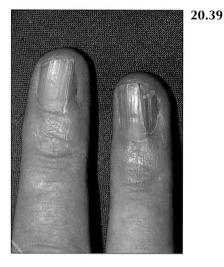

20.39

20.39 Pterygium. Fusion of the posterior nailfold and nail plate due to lichen planus.

Nailfold telangiectasia

In this condition, the blood supply to the posterior nailfolds is essentially the same as that at other skin sites except that the capillary loops run parallel rather than vertical to the surface. Capillaries in the thin posterior nailfold skin are thus easily visible and can be inspected using an ophthalmoscope. The nailfold capillaries are most evident in the ring finger. Normal nailfold capillaries can usually just be seen as uniform loops of similar-thickness capillaries arranged in rows (**20.40**). Alterations to this pattern occur in connective tissue diseases.

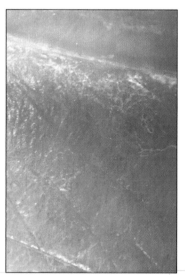

20.40

20.40 Normal nailfold capillaries. These are just visible as tiny capillary loops, uniformly distributed across the posterior nailfold.

Similar capillary changes are seen in dermatomyositis (**20.41**, **20.42**) and systemic sclerosis (**20.43**, **20.44**) (scleroderma), although the changes are most obvious in dermatomyositis. Capillaries disappear, leaving gaps in the normally uniform rows of regular loops. Some remaining capillary loops become dilated and deformed, producing the giant capillary loops (**20.41**). In dermatomyositis, changes also occur on the cuticles, which become ragged, and the posterior nailfolds become red and thickened (**20.42**). It is these changes that seem to be most helpful in making a diagnosis, rather than the shape of the nailfold capillaries.

In lupus erythematosus, the capillaries lose the normal tight loop shape and become irregular or tortuous, but are not dilated.

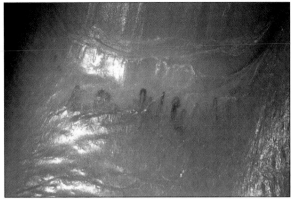

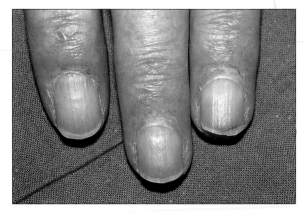

20.41, 20.42 Nailfold capillary changes in dermatomyositis. There are several giant capillary loops and segments without capillaries (**20.41**). The posterior nailfolds are swollen and erythematous, and the cuticles long and ragged (**20.42**) (**20.41** *courtesy of Dr Colin Munro*).

20.43

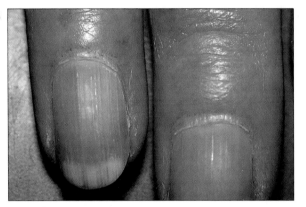

20.44

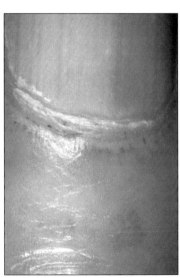

20.43, 20.44 Nailfold capillary changes in systemic sclerosis. The capillaries are dilated and irregularly distributed along the posterior nailfold (**20.43**). Remnants of old nailfold capillaries appear as linear fragments of altered blood visible in the cuticles. Note also the new vessel formation on the terminal phalanx at the site of a mat-like telangiectasia (**20.44**). Same patient as shown in **12.33**.

Paronychia

The term paronychia is used to describe inflammation of the nailfolds. **Acute paronychia** results in redness, swelling, tenderness and pustules of the lateral and posterior nailfold (**20.45**). Infection of the soft tissue, usually by *Staphylococcus aureus*, is the commonest cause. Secondary nail dystrophy with transverse ridging is common.

Herpes simplex infection of the nailfolds can also appear rapidly, but is characterised by grouped vesicles which may be pustular. Acute paronychia rarely progresses to chronic paronychia.

Chronic paronychia is insidious in onset. The nailfold is red and swollen but not particularly painful. There is loss of cuticle and a gap between the nail plate and fold (**20.46**). In some cases, cheesy white material can be squeezed from the posterior nailfold. *Candida albicans*, *Klebsiella* species and proteus organisms are commonly present (**Table 20.8**).

20.45

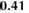

20.45 Acute paronychia. There is swelling and redness of the nailfold. Note that the cuticle is intact.

20.46

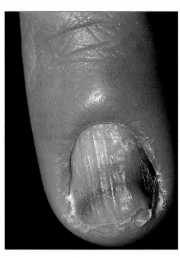

Table 20.8 Causes of acute and chronic paronychia.

Acute	
Bacterial	*Staphylococcus. aureus* *Streptococcus pyogenes*
Viral	Herpes simplex (nurses and dentists)
Chronic[*]	
Candida albicans	Occupational: barmaids, cooks, diabetics, dentists. Chronic cutaneous candidiasis usually only affects the nail plate Hypoparathyroidism
Mycobacterium tuberculosis	Occupational: mortuary attendants and pathologists

[*]Consider the possibility of melanoma or carcinoma in solitary nail involvement, and pustular psoriasis if several nails are involved.

20.46 Chronic paronychia. There is swelling and redness of the posterior and lateral nailfold, loss of cuticles and associated mild nail plate dystrophy. Thick cheesy white material may be squeezed from the junction between the nail plate and nail bed. The lesion is usually surprisingly pain free.

Scaling and hyperkeratosis of the nailfolds

Scaling and hyperkeratosis of the nailfolds are usually caused by psoriasis. Redness and peeling of the nailfold skin are also a feature of zinc deficiency (**20.47**) and acrokeratosis paraneoplastica (**20.48**). The latter is a cutaneous manifestation of internal malignancy seen in men with solid tumours of the upper gastrointestinal or respiratory tract. In this rare condition, there is hyperkeratosis and flaking of the nail plate, and ultimately complete nail loss with only fragments of crumbling nail plate attached to the red nail bed.

20.47

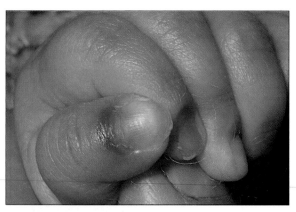

20.48

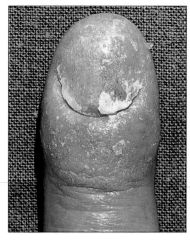

20.47 Zinc deficiency in a breast-fed premature infant. There was erythema and scaling of the nailfolds of the thumb, index and middle fingers of both hands. Other features are shown in **5.17, 5.18**. The clinical features are the same as for acrodermatitis enteropathica, although the zinc deficiency is due to inadequate intake rather than malabsorption. Premature infants are zinc deficient, and breast milk does not contain sufficient excess of zinc to compensate. (From Munro, C. S. *et al.* (1989). Symptomatic zinc deficiency in breast-fed premature infants. *Brit. J. Dermatol.,* **121**: 773 (2c). Published by Blackwell Scientific Publications Ltd and used with permission.)

20.48 Acrokeratosis paraneoplastica (Basex syndrome). There is virtually a complete loss of the nail plate, with only remnants attached to the nail bed, in this elderly man with a carcinoma of the larynx.

Discolouration of the nailfolds

Uneven macular pigmentation of posterior and lateral nailfolds occurs in acral lentiginous melanoma (**20.63, 20.64**). If the tumour is situated in the nail matrix an associated pigmented band will also be present (Hutchinson's sign).

Defects of the nail bed

Onycholysis

Detachment of the nail from the nail bed is common and there are a variety of causes (**Table 20.9**).

Table 20.9 Common causes of onycholysis.

Dermatological	Psoriasis (**20.50**)
Systemic	Thyrotoxicosis, chronic ischaemia (**20.22**) Yellow nail syndrome (**20.61**)
Trauma	Direct injury, excessive manicuring
Drug-induced	Retinoids, cytotoxics
Photo-onycholysis	Usually fingernails only—tetracyclines, thiazides, benoxaprofen, chlorpromazine
Infection	Dermatophyte, candida (**20.37**), viral warts
Chemical irritants	Hot soapy water immersion, false nails, nail varnish remover, solvent and oil injury (**20.14**)
Idiopathic	Usually women with long nails (? traumatic)

Salmon patches

Salmon pink patches on the nail bed visible through the nail plate are due to psoriasis in the nail bed (**20.49**). This can be a helpful diagnostic feature, sometimes called the oil drop sign, since it enables psoriatic and fungal nail dystrophy to be distinguished clinically. The appearance may be seen in isolation, but usually occurs just proximal to an area of psoriatic onycholysis. Attempts to remove debris and keratinous scale from the onycholytic psoriatic nail may result in trauma of the nail bed and further extension of the nail bed psoriasis. Psoriatic nails should be kept short and only cleaned with a soft nail brush.

20.49

20.49 Onycholysis and salmon patches (*photo courtesy of Dr David de Berker*).

Splinter haemorrhages

Splinter haemorrhages are purpuric lesions which develop a linear shape because the nail bed capillaries run along the well-defined folds that exist in the nail bed. The most frequent cause of splinter haemorrhages is trauma (**20.50**), but the most important causes are related to embolic and vasculitic disorders, such as subacute bacterial endocarditis (**20.51**). In this disorder there may be evidence of vasculitis elsewhere, especially in the finger pulps (Osler's nodes—**20.52**) and the palms and soles (Janeway's lesions).

20.50

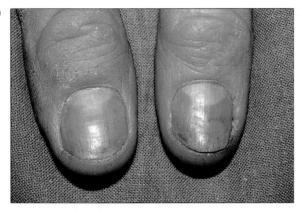

20.50 Traumatic splinter haemorrhages.

20.51

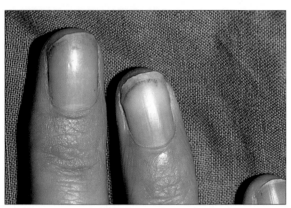

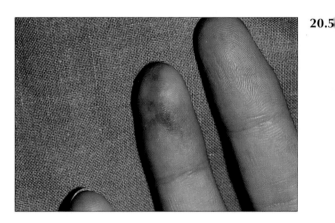

20.5

20.51, 20.52 Splinter haemorrhages and Osler's nodes. The patient presented with embolic cerebrovascular disease. The splinter haemorrhages are visible along the distal margin of the nail plate (**20.51**). The Osler's node occurred as a circumscribed indurated tender red area of the finger pulp (**20.52**).

Tumours associated with the nail

Subungual heloma or corn

A subungual heloma or corn appears as a painful dark spot under the nail and may produce splitting or elevation of the nail tip. It must be distinguished from a subungual melanoma.

Subungual exostosis

Subungual exostoses are out-growths of normal bone or calcified cartilage from the terminal phalanx of any digit. They may be confused with subungual solitary warts, but can be distinguished by the characteristic X-ray changes (**20.53**, *see also* **9.12, 9.13**).

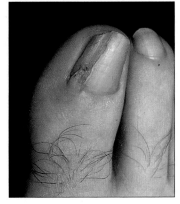

20.53

20.53 Subungual exostosis. There is a small bony spicule protruding from the terminal phalanx, which can be demonstrated on X-ray (*see* **9.13**). Unlike subungual warts, they are solitary, hard and painful.

Koenen's tumours

Periungual fibrokeratoma occurs in 50% of patients with tuberous sclerosis (**20.54**), but it also occurs as solitary sporadic lesions (**20.55**). It may cause longitudinal ridging or guttering of the nail plate, due to pressure on the matrix.

Acquired periungual fibrokeratoma presents as solitary benign nodule with a hyperkeratotic tip arising out of the posterior nailfold, and virtually always causing guttering of the nail plate (**20.55**). By contrast, the periungal fibromas in tuberous sclerosis are multiple and fleshy.

20.54

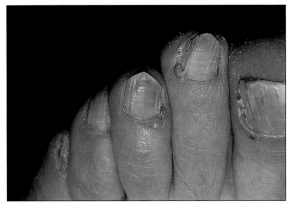

20.55

20.54 Koenen's tumours in tuberous sclerosis. Multiple fleshy periungual fibrokeratomas in a patient with tuberous sclerosis, who was the mother of the patient shown in **3.21**. Approximately 30% of patients with tuberous sclerosis have fibrokeratomas.

20.55 Acquired periungual fibro-keratoma. There is obvious nail guttering produced by this solitary fibrokeratoma arising in otherwise healthy individuals. Tuberous sclerosis must be excluded by the absence of other features. Acquired fibrokeratoma is usually solitary, produces a well-formed nail gutter, and is surmounted by a little hyperkeratotic tip.

Pyogenic granuloma

20.56

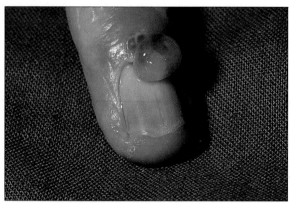

Pyogenic granuloma of the finger presents as an extremely vascular tumour of recent onset (*see* **10.53**), usually arising after minor trauma, and may have a well-defined collar of normal skin—the acorn cup sign (*see* **9.15**). Pyogenic granulomas may arise on the proximal nailfold (**20.56**). When they arise on the nail bed they perforate the nail plate and must be distinguished histologically from amelanotic melanomas.

20.56 Pyogenic granuloma. There is a fleshy vascular tumour on the posterior nailfold, producing a groove in the nail plate.

Glomus tumour

Glomus bodies are neurovascular arteriovenous anastomoses, of which there are multiple on the finger ends. In response to cold, glomus bodies dilate, whereas arterioles constrict, so that blood supply to digits is preserved in cold weather. Benign tumours of glomus bodies may appear under the nail plate, where they produce intolerable pulsating or spontaneous pain made worse by minor trauma. The tumour can be seen through the nail plate as a bluish patch up to 10 mm in diameter, but the changes are usually unimpressive until an attempt is made to squeeze the nail plate (**20.57, 20.58**). Nail plate ridging may be present.

20.57

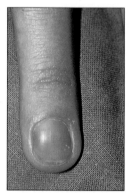

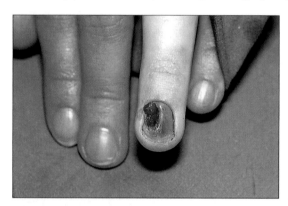

20.58

20.57, 20.58 Glomus tumour and intra-operative appearance. There was relatively little to see before nail removal (**20.57**), although the finger end was exquisitely painful. After removal of the nail plate and excision of the underlying bluish dome of the glomus, the tumour was also found to be extending under the posterior and lateral nailfolds (**20.58**). The soft pinkish tumour tissue has been scooped out of the excision and is resting on the nail bed. Note the white finger due to the tourniquet.

Myxoid cysts

Myxoid cysts (digital mucous cysts) are soft cystic dome-shaped skin-covered papules, usually found on the posterior nailfold of the finger or toe (*see* **14.31**); pressure on the underlying nail plate may cause guttering. Puncture of the cyst results in release of a gelatinous material. When methylene blue dye is injected into the distal interphalangeal joint, it also enters the cyst, demonstrating that virtually all myxoid cysts are connected to the joint and supports the theory that myxoid cysts are derived from extruded joint fluid.

Periungual warts

Periungual warts (**20.59**) are common. Posterior nailfold warts occur in children who bite or chew their fingers, in which case the virus is often spread to the lips. Subungual warts can become impossible to treat without removal of the nail plate and extensive diathermy or carbon dioxide laser destruction of the affected area.

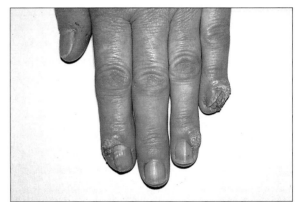
20.59

20.59 Periungual warts. Multiple warts on the fingertips. On the little finger, the nail plate is becoming lifted up by warts growing into the nail bed. Notice the changes produced by chewing the nailfolds present on the thumb. Persistent finger tip warts usually occur only in nail biters and finger chewers who constantly damage their finger ends, providing more sites for the virus to penetrate.

Carcinoma of the fingertip

Squamous carcinoma or Bowen's disease of a digit (**20.60**) may present as chronic paronychia, destruction of the nail or subungual keratosis. A biopsy should be performed if doubt exists.

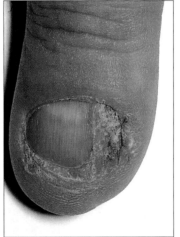
20.60

20.60 Bowen's disease of the finger. There is destruction of half of the nail plate, which is replaced by hyperkeratotic tumour (*photo courtesy of Dr Peter Farr*).

Nail colour changes and pigmented streaks

There are multiple causes of nail colour change. Most are incidental features and rarely present diagnostic difficulty. Complete lists are included in specialist textbooks. Some of the common types of colour change are given in **Tables 20.10** and **20.11**.

Table 20.10 Common causes of pigmented streaks.

- **Benign naevus of the matrix**
- **Physiological in black skin (20.6)**
- **Traumatic**
- **Laugier–Hunziker syndrome**
  With lentigines of the lips, mouth and hands (**20.70, 20.71**)
- **Systemic disease**
  Addison's disease, post-adrenalectomy for Cushing's disease
- **Drugs**
  Mepacrine (**20.67**), chemotherapeutic drugs including busulphan, cyclophosphamide
- **Melanoma (20.63–20.66)**

Table 20.11 Causes of other nail colour changes.

Generalised whitening of the nail	Cirrhosis, chronic hypoalbuminaemia, renal failure, etc. (**20.68**)
Proximal half white	Half and half nails occur in 10% of patients with chronic renal failure—it does not correspond to the degree of renal impairment (**20.69**)
Other colours	Blue—drugs, e.g. antimalarials (**20.67**), minocycline (*see* **3.3**) Yellow—yellow nail syndrome (**20.61**) Green—pseudomonas infections (**20.62**) Tan—scopulariopsis infection

20.61

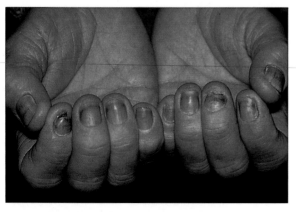

20.61 Yellow nail syndrome finger. All the nails are yellowish and thickened. There were identical changes in the toenails.

20.62 Pseudomonas infection. There is onycholysis and a green colour to the nail plate. Pseudomonas was cultured from nail clippings.

20.62

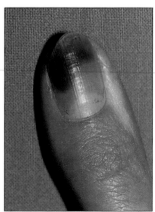

Pigmented streaks

Eighty per cent of Afro-Carribeans have pigmented streaks in the fingernails (**20.6**). The appearance of pigmented streaks in whites suggests the development of a subungual melanoma, but there are many other causes (**Table 20.10**).

Features that are suggestive of melanoma include:

- Pigmented streak is wider proximally than distally—this occurs if the tumour width expands faster than the time taken for the nail to grow from the tumour to the free nail edge.
- Pigment spread from the nail plate onto the posterior nailfold—Hutchinson's sign (**20.63, 20.64**).
- Nail destruction, although this also occurs in subungual corn, pyogenic granuloma and fungal infections, etc.

Note that the origin of a pigmented streak may be obscured by the nail plate and can only be demonstrated surgically (**20.65, 20.66**).

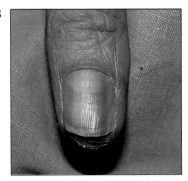

20.63

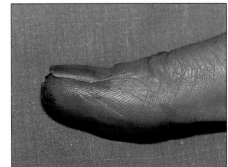

20.64

20.63, 20.64 Acral lentiginous melanoma *in situ*. There is a faint pigment band on the nail plate (**20.63**); pigment spread onto the lateral nailfold and finger end (Hutchinson's sign) is most evident in the lateral view (**20.64**).

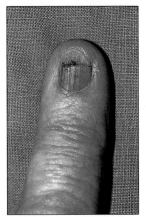

20.65

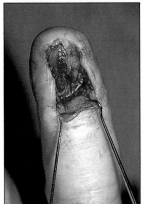

20.66

20.65, 20.66 Acral lentiginous melanoma. The nail is slightly pigmented (**20.65**), although a previous biopsy has obscured this. The nail plate was thickened and smaller than the equivalent nail on the other hand. After nail plate removal pigmentation of the nail bed can be clearly seen (**20.66**).

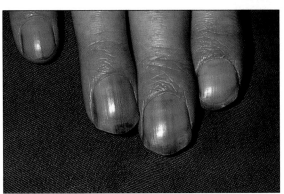

20.67

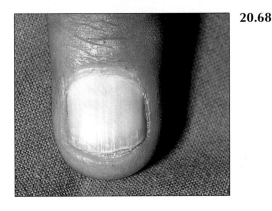

20.68

20.67 Nail pigmentation due to mepacrine. Grey-brown pigmented bands associated with mepacrine treatment for discoid lupus erythematosus.

20.68 Generalised leukonychia in renal failure. Loss of lunula and sparing of the onychodermal band of Terry.

20.69

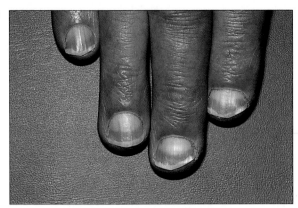

20.69 Half and half nails. Half and half nails in a patient with rheumatoid disease and chronic renal failure. The proximal portion is white and the distal red, pink or brown. This condition occurs in approximately 10% of patients with chronic renal failure. The level and extent of colour change are not related to the severity of the uraemia.

20.70

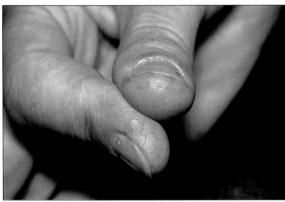

20.71

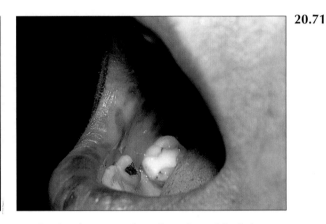

20.70, 20.71 Laugier–Hunziker syndrome. This is a benign cause of isolated pigmented streaks in the nail bed; they are just visible on the nail (**20.70**). Pigment spread onto the nailfolds may occur. Other characteristic features include brown macules on the lips and buccal mucosa (**20.71**), and pigmented macules on the fingertips (**20.70**).

Bibliography

General Reading

T. B. Fitzpatrick, A. Z. Eisen, K. Wolff, I. M. Freedburg & K. F. Austen (1987). *Dermatology in General Medicine*, 3rd edn, McGraw-Hill Inc., New York.

R. H. Champion, J. L. Burton & F. J. B. Ebling (eds) (1992). *Rook, Wilkinson & Ebling Textbook of Dermatology*, 5th edn, edited by R. H. Champion, J. L. Burton & F. J. G. Ebling, Blackwell Scientific Publications, Oxford.

T. P. Habif (1990). *Clinical Dermatology. A color guide to diagnosis and therapy,* 2nd edition, Mosby, St Louis.

O. Braun-Falco, G. Plewig, H. H. Wolff & R. K. Winkelmann (1991). *Dermatology,* 3rd revised edn, Springer-Verlag, Berlin.

2. Shapes and Patterns of Lesions

R. Happle (1985). Lyonisation and the lines of Blaschko. *Hum. Genet.* **70**: 200–206.

C. F. Farthing, R.C.D. Staughton J. I. Harper, *et. al. (1986).* Papuloerythroderma: a further case with the deck chair sign. *Dermatologica* **172**: 65–66.

3. Colours, Hyperpigmentation, Hypopigmentation

J.-P. Ortonne, D. B. Mosher & T. B. Fitzpatrick (1983). *Vitiligo and other hypomelanoses of hair and skin,* Plenum Medical Book Company, New York.

C. S. Fulk (1984). Primary disorders of hyperpigmentation. *J. Am. Acad. Dermatol.* **10**: 1–16.

G. B. Colver, P. S. Mortimer, P. R. Millard, R. P. R. Dawber & T. J. Ryan (1987). The 'Dirty neck' a reticulate pigmentation in atopics. *Clin. Exper. Dermatol.* **12**: 1–4.

J. A. Hud, J. B. Cohen, J. M. Wagner & P. D. Crus (1992). Prevalence and significance of acanthosis nigricans in an adult obese population. *Arch. Dermatol.* **128**: 941–944.

4. Elicitation of Physical Signs

A. Clarke & J. Burn (1991). Sweat testing to identify female carriers of X-linked hypohidrotic ectodermal dysplasia. *J. Med. Genet.* **28**: 330–333.

6. Normal Variants and Common Anomalies

V. J. Selmanowitz & J. M. Krivo (1975). Pigmentary demarcation lines. *Brit. J. Dermatol.* **93**: 371–377.

F. Nürnberger & G. Müller (1978). So Called Cellulite: An Inventive Disease. *J. Dermatol. Surg. Oncol.* **4**: 221–229.

T. Lewis (1927). *The Blood Vessels of the Human Skin and their Responses*, Shaw & Sons Ltd, London.

N. Kirkham, *et. al.* (1989). Diagonal ear lobe creases and fatal cardiovascular disease: a necropsy study. *Brit. Heart J.* **61**: 361–364.

7. Scale and Crust

Y. Paramsothy & C. M. Lawrence (1987). Tin tack sign in localised pemphigus foliaceus. *Brit. J. Dermatol.* **116**: 127–129.

M. R. Caro & F. E. Senear (1947). Psoriasis of the hands: non-pustular type. *Arch. Dermatol. Syphilol.* **56**: 629–632.

8. Plaques

J. D. Bernhard (1990). Auspitz sign is not sensitive or specific for psoriasis. *J. Amer. Acad. Dermatol.* **22**: 1079–1081.

11. Macular and Maculopapular Rashes

H. M. Goodyear, *et. al.* (1991). Acute infectious erythemas in children: a clinico-microbiological study. *Brit. J. Dermatol.* **124**: 433–438.

C. Bialecki , H. M. Feder & J. M. Grant-Kels (1989). The six classic childhood exanthems; a review and update. *J. Am. Acad. Dermatol.* **21**: 891–903.

12. Textural Changes in Skin

J. L. Burton (1982). Thick skin and stiff joints in insulin dependent diabetes mellitus. *Brit. J. Dermatol.* **106**: 369–371.

A. C. Hartley (1986). Finger pebbles: a common finding in diabetes mellitus. *J. Am. Acad. Dermatol.* **14**: 612–617.

13. Ulcers

C. Moss & P. Ince (1987). Anhidrotic and achromians lesions in incontinentia pigmenti. *Brit. J. Dermtol.* **116**: 839–849.

G. Asboe-Hansen (1960). Blister spread induced by finger pressure, a diagnostic sign in pemphigus. *J. Invest. Dermatol.* **34**: 5–9.

D. S. Feingold (1982). Gangrenous and Crepitant Cellulitis. *J. Am. Acad. Dermatol.* **6**: 289–299.

17. Weals

B. M. Czarnetzki (1986). *Urticaria.* Springer-Verlag, Berlin.

18. Erythema and Vascular Disorders

W. W. Piette & M. S. Stone (1989). A cutaneous sign of IgA-associated small dermal vessel leukocytoclastic vasculitis in adults (Henoch–Schönlein purpura). *Arch. Dermatol.* **125**: 53–56.

N. H. Cox & W. D. Paterson (1991). Angioma serpiginosum: a simulator of purpura. *Postgrad. Med. J.* **67**: 1065–1066.

J. V. Hirschmann, G. J. Raugi (1992). Dermatologic features of the superior vena cava syndrome. *Arch. Dermatol.* **128**: 953–956.

19. Hair

S. Shuster (1984). 'Coudability': a new physical sign of alopecia areata. *Brit. J. Dermatol.* **111**: 629.

Leonard C. Sperling (1991). Hair anatomy for the clinician. *J. Am. Acad. Dermatol.* **25**: 1–17.

Diseases of the Hair and Scalp, 2nd edn (1991). Edited by A. Rook & R. P. R. Dawber, Blackwell Scientific Publications, Oxford.

20. Nails

Diseases of the Nail and their Management (1984). Edited by R. Baran & R. P. R. Dawber, Blackwell Scientific Publications, Oxford.

W. Minkin & N. B. Rabhan (1982). Office nailfold capillary microscopy using an ophthalmoscope. *J. Am. Acad. Dermatol.* **7**: 190–193.

R. Baran (1979). Longitudinal melanotic streaks as a clue to Laugier–Hunziker syndrome. *Arch. Dermatol.* **115**: 1448–1449.

LOTRISONE®

brand of clotrimazole
and betamethasone
dipropionate

Cream, USP

For Dermatologic Use Only –
Not for Ophthalmic Use

DESCRIPTION LOTRISONE Cream contains a combination of clotrimazole, USP, a synthetic antifungal agent, and betamethasone dipropionate, USP, a synthetic corticosteroid, for dermatologic use.

Chemically, clotrimazole is 1-(o-Chloro-α,α-diphenylbenzyl) imidazole, with the empirical formula $C_{22}H_{17}ClN_2$, a molecular weight of 344.8, and the following structural formula:

Clotrimazole is an odorless, white crystalline powder, insoluble in water and soluble in ethanol.

Betamethasone dipropionate has the chemical name 9-Fluoro-11ß,17,21-trihydroxy-16ß-methylpregna-1, 4-diene-3,20-dione 17,21-dipropionate, with the empirical formula $C_{28}H_{37}FO_7$, a molecular weight of 504.6, and the following structural formula:

Betamethasone dipropionate is a white to creamy white, odorless crystalline powder, insoluble in water.

Each gram of LOTRISONE Cream contains 10.0 mg clotrimazole, USP and 0.64 mg betamethasone dipropionate, USP (equivalent to 0.5 mg betamethasone), in a hydrophilic emollient cream consisting of purified water, mineral oil, white petrolatum, cetearyl alcohol, ceteareth-30, propylene glycol, sodium phosphate monobasic, and phosphoric acid; benzyl alcohol as preservative.

LOTRISONE is a smooth, uniform, white to off-white cream.

CLINICAL PHARMACOLOGY

Clotrimazole

Clotrimazole is a broad-spectrum, antifungal agent that is used for the treatment of dermal infections caused by various species of pathogenic dermatophytes, yeasts, and *Malassezia furfur*. The primary action of clotrimazole is against dividing and growing organisms.

In vitro, clotrimazole exhibits fungistatic and fungicidal activity against isolates of *Trichophyton rubrum, Trichophyton mentagrophytes, Epidermophyton floccosum,* and *Microsporum canis*. In general, the *in vitro* activity of clotrimazole corresponds to that of tolnaftate and griseofulvin against the mycelia of dermatophytes (*Trichophyton, Microsporum,* and *Epidermophyton*).

In vivo studies in guinea pigs infected with *Trichophyton mentagrophytes* have shown no measurable loss of clotrimazole activity due to combination with betamethasone dipropionate.

Strains of fungi having a natural resistance to clotrimazole have not been reported.

No single-step or multiple-step resistance to clotrimazole has developed during successive passages of *Trichophyton mentagrophytes*.

In studies of the mechanism of action in fungal cultures, the minimum fungicidal concentration of clotrimazole caused leakage of intracellular phosphorous compounds into the ambient medium with concomitant breakdown of cellular nucleic acids, and accelerated potassium efflux. Both of these events began rapidly and extensively after addition of the drug to the cultures.

Clotrimazole appears to be minimally absorbed following topical application to the skin. Six hours after the application of radioactive clotrimazole 1% cream and 1% solution onto intact and acutely inflamed skin, the concentration of clotrimazole varied from 100 mcg/cm³ in the stratum corneum, to 0.5 to 1 mcg/cm³ in the stratum reticulare, and 0.1 mcg/cm³ in the subcutis. No measurable amount of radioactivity (<0.001 mcg/mL) was found in the serum within 48 hours after application under occlusive dressing of 0.5 mL of the solution or 0.8 g of the cream.

Betamethasone dipropionate

Betamethasone dipropionate, a corticosteroid, is effective in the treatment of corticosteroid-responsive dermatoses primarily because of its anti-inflammatory, anti-pruritic, and vasoconstrictive actions. However, while the physiologic, pharmacologic, and clinical effects of corticosteroids are well known, the exact mechanisms of their actions in each disease are uncertain. Betamethasone dipropionate, a corticosteroid, has been shown to have topical (dermatologic) and systemic pharmacologic and metabolic effects characteristic of this class of drugs.

Pharmacokinetics The extent of percutaneous absorption of topical corticosteroids is determined by many factors including the vehicle, the integrity of the epidermal barrier, and the use of occlusive dressings. (See **DOSAGE AND ADMINIS-TRATION** section.)

Topical corticosteroids can be absorbed from normal intact skin. Inflammation and/or other disease processes in the skin increase percutaneous absorption. Occlusive dressings substantially increase the percutaneous absorption of topical corticosteroids. (See **DOSAGE AND ADMINISTRATION** section.)

Once absorbed through the skin, topical corticosteroids are handled through pharmacokinetic pathways similar to systemically administered corticosteroids. Corticosteroids are bound to plasma proteins in varying degrees. Corticosteroids are metabolized primarily in the liver and are then excreted by the kidneys. Some of the topical corticosteroids and their metabolites are also excreted into the bile.

Clotrimazole and betamethasone dipropionate

In clinical studies of tinea corporis, tinea cruris, and tinea pedis, patients treated with LOTRISONE Cream showed a better clinical response at the first return visit than patients treated with clotrimazole cream. In tinea corporis and tinea cruris, the patient returned 3 days after starting treatment, and in tinea pedis, after 1 week. Mycological cure rates observed in patients treated with LOTRISONE Cream were as good as or better than in those patients treated with clotrimazole cream.

In these same clinical studies, patients treated with LOTRISONE Cream showed statistically significantly better clinical responses and mycological cure rates when compared with patients treated with betamethasone dipropionate cream.

INDICATIONS AND USAGE LOTRISONE Cream is indicated for the topical treatment of the following dermal infections: tinea pedis, tinea cruris, and tinea corporis due to *Trichophyton rubrum, Trichophyton mentagrophytes, Epidermophyton floccosum,* and *Microsporum canis*.

CONTRAINDICATIONS LOTRISONE Cream is contraindicated in patients who are sensitive to clotrimazole, betamethasone dipropionate, other corticosteroids or imidazoles, or to any ingredient in this preparation.

PRECAUTIONS General Systemic absorption of topical corticosteroids has produced reversible hypothalamic-pituitary-adrenal (HPA) axis suppression, manifestations of Cushing's syndrome, hyperglycemia, and glucosuria in some patients.

Conditions which augment systemic absorption include the application of the more potent steroids, use over large surface areas, prolonged use, and the addition of occlusive dressings. (See **DOSAGE AND ADMINISTRATION** section.)

Therefore, patients receiving a large dose of a potent topical steroid applied to a large surface area should be evaluated periodically for evidence of HPA axis suppression by using the urinary free cortisol and ACTH stimulation tests. If HPA axis suppression is noted, an attempt should be made to withdraw the drug, to reduce the frequency of application, or to substitute a less potent steroid.

Recovery of HPA axis function is generally prompt and complete upon discontinuation of the drug. Infrequently, signs and symptoms of steroid withdrawal may occur, requiring supplemental systemic corticosteroids.

Children may absorb proportionally larger amounts of topical corticosteroids and thus be more susceptible to systemic toxicity. (See **PRECAUTIONS – Pediatric Use**.)

If irritation or hypersensitivity develops with the use of LOTRISONE Cream, treatment should be discontinued and appropriate therapy instituted.

LOTRISONE®

brand of clotrimazole
and betamethasone
dipropionate

Cream, USP

**For Dermatologic Use Only –
Not for Ophthalmic Use**

Information for Patients Patients using LOTRISONE Cream should receive the following information and instructions:
1. This medication is to be used as directed by the physician. It is for external use only. Avoid contact with the eyes.
2. The medication is to be used for the full prescribed treatment time, even though the symptoms may have improved. Notify the physician if there is no improvement after 1 week of treatment for tinea cruris or tinea corporis, or after 2 weeks for tinea pedis.
3. Patients should be advised not to use this medication for any disorder other than for which it was prescribed.
4. The treated skin areas should not be bandaged or otherwise covered or wrapped as to be occluded. (See **DOSAGE AND ADMINISTRATION** section.)
5. When using this medication in the groin area, patients should be advised to use the medication for 2 weeks only, and to apply the cream sparingly. The physician should be notified if the condition persists after 2 weeks. Patients should also be advised to wear loose fitting clothing. (See **DOSAGE AND ADMINISTRATION** section.)
6. Patients should report any signs of local adverse reactions.
7. Patients should avoid sources of infection or reinfection.

Laboratory Tests If there is a lack of response to LOTRISONE Cream, appropriate microbiological studies should be repeated to confirm the diagnosis and rule out other pathogens before instituting another course of antimycotic therapy.

The following tests may be helpful in evaluating HPA axis suppression due to the corticosteroid component:

Urinary free cortisol test

ACTH stimulation test

Carcinogenesis, Mutagenesis, Impairment of Fertility There are no animal or laboratory studies with the combination clotrimazole and betamethasone dipropionate to evaluate carcinogenesis, mutagenesis, or impairment of fertility.

An 18-month oral dosing study with clotrimazole in rats has not revealed any carcinogenic effect.

In tests for mutagenesis, chromosomes of the spermatophores of Chinese hamsters which had been exposed to clotrimazole were examined for structural changes during the metaphase. Prior to testing, the hamsters had received five oral clotrimazole doses of 100 mg/kg body weight. The results of this study showed that clotrimazole had no mutagenic effect.

Pregnancy Category C There have been no teratogenic studies performed with the combination clotrimazole and betamethasone dipropionate.

Studies in pregnant rats with intravaginal doses up to 100 mg/kg have revealed no evidence of harm to the fetus due to clotrimazole.

High oral doses of clotrimazole in rats and mice ranging from 50 to 120 mg/kg resulted in embryotoxicity (possibly secondary to maternal toxicity), impairment of mating, decreased litter size and number of viable young and decreased pup survival to weaning. However, clotrimazole was not teratogenic in mice, rabbits, and rats at oral doses up to 200, 180, and 100 mg/kg, respectively. Oral absorption in the rat amounts to approximately 90% of the administered dose.

Corticosteroids are generally teratogenic in laboratory animals when administered systemically at relatively low dosage levels. The more potent corticosteroids have been shown to be teratogenic after dermal application in laboratory animals.

There are no adequate and well-controlled studies in pregnant women on teratogenic effects from a topically applied combination of clotrimazole and betamethasone dipropionate. Therefore, LOTRISONE Cream should be used during pregnancy only if the potential benefit justifies the potential risk to the fetus.

Drugs containing corticosteroids should not be used extensively on pregnant patients, in large amounts, or for prolonged periods of time.

Nursing Mothers It is not known whether this drug is excreted in human milk. Because many drugs are excreted in human milk, caution should be exercised when LOTRISONE Cream is used by a nursing woman.

Pediatric Use Safety and effectiveness in children below the age of 12 have not been established with LOTRISONE Cream.

Pediatric patients may demonstrate greater susceptibility to topical corticosteroid-induced HPA axis suppression and Cushing's syndrome than mature patients because of a larger skin surface area to body weight ratio.

Hypothalamic-pituitary-adrenal (HPA) axis suppression, Cushing's syndrome, and intracranial hypertension have been reported in children receiving topical corticosteroids. Manifestations of adrenal suppression in children include linear growth retardation, delayed weight gain, low plasma cortisol levels, and absence of response to ACTH stimulation. Manifestations of intracranial hypertension include bulging fontanelles, headaches, and bilateral papilledema.

Administration of topical dermatologics containing a corticosteroid to children should be limited to the least amount compatible with an effective therapeutic regimen. Chronic corticosteroid therapy may interfere with the growth and development of children.

The use of LOTRISONE Cream in diaper dermatitis is not recommended.

ADVERSE REACTIONS The following adverse reactions have been reported in connection with the use of LOTRISONE Cream: paresthesia in 5 of 270 patients, maculopapular rash, edema, and secondary infection, each in 1 of 270 patients.

Adverse reactions reported with the use of clotrimazole are as follows: erythema, stinging, blistering, peeling, edema, pruritus, urticaria, and general irritation of the skin.

The following local adverse reactions are reported infrequently when topical corticosteroids are used as recommended. These reactions are listed in an approximate decreasing order of occurrence: burning, itching, irritation, dryness, folliculitis, hypertrichosis, acneiform eruptions, hypopigmentation, perioral dermatitis, allergic contact dermatitis, maceration of the skin, secondary infection, skin atrophy, striae, and miliaria.

OVERDOSAGE Acute overdosage with topical application of LOTRISONE Cream is unlikely and would not be expected to lead to a life-threatening situation.

Topically applied corticosteroids can be absorbed in sufficient amounts to produce systemic effects. (See **PRECAUTIONS**.)

DOSAGE AND ADMINISTRATION Gently massage sufficient LOTRISONE Cream into the affected and surrounding skin areas twice a day, in the morning and evening, for 2 weeks in tinea cruris and tinea corporis and for 4 weeks in tinea pedis. The use of LOTRISONE Cream for longer than 4 weeks is not recommended.

Clinical improvement, with relief of erythema and pruritus, usually occurs within 3 to 5 days of treatment. If a patient with tinea cruris or tinea corporis shows no clinical improvement after 1 week of treatment with LOTRISONE Cream, the diagnosis should be reviewed. In tinea pedis, the treatment should be applied for 2 weeks prior to making that decision.

Treatment with LOTRISONE Cream should be discontinued if the condition persists after 2 weeks in tinea cruris and tinea corporis, and after 4 weeks in tinea pedis. Alternate therapy may then be instituted with LOTRIMIN Cream, a product containing an antifungal only.

LOTRISONE Cream should not be used with occlusive dressings.

HOW SUPPLIED LOTRISONE Cream is supplied in 15-gram (NDC 0085-0924-01) and 45-gram tubes (NDC 0085-0924-02); boxes of one.

Store between 2° and 30°C (36° and 86°F).

Schering **/KEY**

Schering Corporation/Key Pharmaceuticals, Inc.
Kenilworth, NJ 07033 USA

Rev. 7/93

13182361

Index

Page numbers in bold print refer to illustrations.